Choate and Usher
Washington, D.C.
January 1985

PROPERTY OF THE
CLINICAL SOCIAL
WORK INSTITUTE

WITH THE EYES OF THE MIND

CREDITS

The authors gratefully acknowledge permission to reprint portions of the following material:

Chapter One
Twemlow, S.W., G.O. Gabbard, and F.C. Jones. "The Out-of-Body Experience: A Phenomenological Typology Based on Questionnaire Responses." *American Journal of Psychiatry* 139(4):450-55, 1982. Portions reprinted with permission.

Chapter Two
Jones, F.C., G.O. Gabbard, and S.W. Twemlow. "Psychological and Demographic Characteristics of Persons Reporting Out-of-Body Experiences." *The Hillside Journal of Clinical Psychiatry* 6(1):105-115, 1984. Copyright 1984 by Human Sciences Press, New York City, New York.

Chapters Three, Four, and Five
Gabbard, G.O., S.W. Twemlow, and F.C. Jones. "Differential Diagnosis of Altered Mind/Body Perception." *Psychiatry* 45(4):361-69, November, 1982. Portions reprinted with permission.

Chapter Seven
Gabbard, G.O., S.W. Twemlow, and F.C. Jones. "Do 'Near-Death Experiences' Occur Only Near Death?" *The Journal of Nervous and Mental Disease* 169(6):374-77, 1981. Portions reprinted with permission.

Chapter Seven
Moody, R. *Life After Life*. Mockingbird Books, Atlanta, 1977, pp. 23-24. Quotation printed with permission.

Chapter Eight
Twemlow, S.W., G.O. Gabbard, and L. Coyne. "A Note on a Multi-Variate Method for the Classification of Preexisting Near-Death Conditions." *Anabiosis* 2:132-39, 1982. Portions reprinted with permission.

Chapter Eight
Twemlow, S.W., and G.O. Gabbard. "The Influence of Demographic/Psychological Factors and Preexisting Conditions on the Near-Death Experience." *Omega*, in press, 1984. Portions reprinted with permission.

WITH THE EYES OF THE MIND _____

An Empirical Analysis
of Out-of-Body States

Foreword by
Stephen Appelbaum

by Glen O. Gabbard
and Stuart W. Twemlow

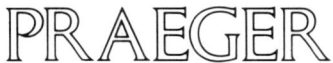

PRAEGER SPECIAL STUDIES • PRAEGER SCIENTIFIC

New York • Philadelphia • Eastbourne, UK
Toronto • Hong Kong • Tokyo • Sydney

Library of Congress Cataloging in Publication Data

Gabbard, Glen O.
  With the eyes of the mind.

  Bibliography: p.
  Includes index.
  1. Astral projection.   2. Death, Apparent.
  3. Mind and body.   I. Twemlow, Stuart W.   II. Title.
  BF1389.A7G32 1984   133.9   84-15914
  ISBN 0-03-068926-0 (alk. paper)

To Matthew, Abigail, Amanda, and Allison

and

To Susan, Stephen, Lee, Megan, Nicholas, and Sarah

Published in 1984 by Praeger Publishers
CBS Educational and Professional Publishing
a Division of CBS Inc.
521 Fifth Avenue, New York, NY 10175 USA

© 1984 by Praeger Publishers

All rights reserved

456789 052 987654321

Printed in the United States of America
on acid-free paper

FOREWORD

Some years back a friend of a friend sent me a report of her experience after being in an auto accident. She wrote that she had watched the aftermath of the collision from a vantage point above it; that she had seen her badly injured body receiving medical treatment. Not long after, I read *Journeys Out of the Body* by Robert Monroe, an autobiographical account of the author's alleged capacity to leave and return to his body. Sealed in a sound-tight room, on a waterbed, with instructions and arcane music piped into my ears through headphones, I tried to duplicate Monroe's feat in his laboratory, but without success. Later, during the hubbub of a convention, Monroe guided me toward what seemed to be at least the beginning of the experience that he described. I became anxious at what was happening to me, which he said was characteristic of those successfully embarking on their first trip.

The easy way to deal with these so-called out-of-body experiences has been to dismiss them as delusions or fakery; they are too remote from usual experience; they violate the laws of traditional physics and of common sense. Developments in the nineteen-sixties and seventies, however, have provided such reports with a welcoming context. That context was spawned by the political, cultural, social ferment of the 1960s and is called variously the counterculture, the consciousness movement, and the human potential movement. With slight modifications this context continues to influence society in the present. Its revisionist trends include the belief that traditional ways of viewing, thinking about, and experiencing reality are limited by the inherent limitations of the senses, and by the sociopsychological needs to know some things and not to know other things. Most people make do with a narrow band of consciousness. Only exceptional people, or ordinary people under exceptional circumstances, are vouchsafed the opportunity to emcompass larger aspects of reality, to transcend the usual limitations of awareness. While many formal religions have always successfully asserted the presence of a supernatural reality, now a wide variety of esoteric disciplines and practices are accorded a comparable consideration: diverse expressions of spirituality, purportedly empirical observations of life after death, past lives, reincarnation, and psychic phenomena. Such openness and freedom from modern Western conceptions of reality are now expressed also in medical and psychological therapies.

In keeping with the counterculture's romantic, naturalistic, anti-intellectual and generally rebellious bent, its adherents eschew and sometimes derogate the scientific method. While freedom from the need for proof facilitates inspirational devotion and encourages creative hypotheses that might otherwise have been inhibited, the exercise of such freedom makes it difficult to know where free-floating fantasy leaves off and possible new knowledge begins. Furthermore, freedom from the need for evidence isolates novel ideas from the possibility of integration with broader social, scientific, and therapeutic cultures. In the midst of the delicious chaos of fresh and seemingly unlimited possibilities for the human spirit, some people, at least, even though intrigued by new versions of reality, have cried out for balance and moderation, for a reasonable respect for discipline and proof. They want methods that both respect the subject matter and advance the possibilities for confidence in the soundness of the new observations.

So far, not many have answered that call. For one thing it requires an unusual sort of person—perhaps even a neurological rarity; those with more or less equal facility with left brain analytical thinking and right brain fancifulness. Rigid and exclusionary educational and professional practices do not help either, nor do the rewards available to those who remain unquestioningly loyal to and exploit traditional forms and practices. Nevertheless, in this book, Drs. Gabbard and Twemlow have answered the call. Trained as psychoanalysts and psychiatrists, imbued with the scientific method, they have long been intrigued with many of the hypotheses of the consciousness movement. They coordinate their openness to, and excitement with, the hypothesis of out-of-body phenomena with the counterculture's tenet of holism (which jibes with enlightened science's recognition of multi-determination and interlocking causes). They enlist in this study psychoanalytic, neurophysiological, and philosophical points of view. In their hands the reader can feel confidently free to learn about, consider, and perhaps thrill to new ways of thinking about himself and the universe.

Stephen A. Appelbaum, Ph.D.

ACKNOWLEDGMENTS

There are many people who have been helpful and supportive to us during the years of this research. Here we can only thank a few of them. First, we wish to acknowledge the participation of Dr. Fowler Jones of the University of Kansas Medical Center, who was a collaborator in the early stages of this work, particularly on the questionnaire survey. Dr. Lolafaye Coyne, Director of the Statistical Laboratory and Associate Director of Hospital Research at The Menninger Foundation, was invaluable in her statistical consultation, as were Mrs. Betty Rosen and Mrs. Beth Thompson, who assisted her. Dr. Robert Ellsworth advised us on the use of the Profiles of Adaption to Life questionnaire. Alice Brand, chief librarian of The Menninger Foundation, deserves special acknowledgment for her help in keeping us abreast of the literature. Dr. William Trussell, Dr. Stephen Appelbaum, and Dr. Tom Matthews assisted in the psychological testing of some of our subjects. We also want to thank several typists who were efficient and patient with us throughout this project: Ms. Jan Bays, Mrs. Faye Schoenfeld, Mrs. Wren Samuel, Ms. Cheryl Zibell, Mrs. Lorene Zibell, Ms. Debi Smith, and Ms. Aleta Pennington. Mr. Duane Callies was most helpful with the artwork. Our research was supported in part by the Department of Psychiatry of the University of Kansas Medical Center, The Menninger Foundation, and the Monroe Institute of Applied Sciences.

Finally, we owe a special debt to our teachers, particularly Dr. Karl Menninger, Chairman of the Board of Trustees of The Menninger Foundation, Dr. Ishak Ramzy, Distinguished Professor of Psychoanalysis, The Menninger Foundation, and Dr. Basil James, formerly Professor of Psychological Medicine, University of Otago Medical School, Dunedin, New Zealand, now Director of Mental Health for New Zealand.

CONTENTS

CREDITS		ii
FOREWORD		v
ACKNOWLEDGMENTS		vii
INTRODUCTION		x

Part I:
The Out-of-Body Experience

One	A Descriptive Typology of the Out-of-Body Experience	3
Two	A Psychological and Demographic Profile of Persons Reporting Out-of-Body Experiences	27

Part II:
Differentiation of the Out-of-Body States

Three	Depersonalization	45
Four	Autoscopy: The Doppelgänger and Beyond	60
Five	Schizophrenic Body Boundary Disturbances	78
Six	"More Real Than a Dream"	94

Part III:
The Near-Death Experience

Seven	An Overview of the Near-Death Experience	123
Eight	The Context of the Near-Death Experience	139
Nine	Three Case Reports of Near-Death Experience in Children	154

Part IV:
Understanding the Out-of-Body Experience

Ten	The Metapsychology of Altered Mind/Body Perception	169
Eleven	Problems of Causation and Meaning in the Out-of-Body Experience	184

Twelve	Psychophysiological Correlates of the Out-of-Body Experience	203
Thirteen	The Mind/Body Trap	222

BIBLIOGRAPHY	241
INDEX	263
ABOUT THE AUTHORS	273

INTRODUCTION

At the end of Book II, Part 3, of Goethe's autobiography, the author makes the following comment: "...then one of the strangest premonitions came over me. I saw myself—not with my real eyes, but with the eyes of the mind—riding horseback toward me on the same road enclothed in a garment such as I had never wore." Goethe's words, some of which contribute to the title of our book, indicate that this experience seemed unusual and bizarre to him. However, such experiences, and variations thereof, are actually quite common. These phenomena may be grouped together under the rubric of altered mind/body perception. They have in common an altered state of consciousness in which there is a subjectively perceived distortion of the normal spatial relationship between the mind and the body. This assortment of "out-of-body" states includes out-of-body experiences, near-death experiences, some forms of depersonalization, and schizophrenic body boundary disturbances. Autoscopy is also discussed in this context because it is frequently confused with these states. This definition excludes dissociative states, such as multiple personality, where the distortion is in the time dimension.

The out-of-body experience may be viewed as the prototype of altered mind/body perception. It serves as a point of reference from which all other "out-of-body" states depart. There has been a trend in the literature to lump together such experiences, resulting in confusion and in the general impression that all forms of altered mind/body perception may be viewed as one monolithic entity. While this book seeks to delineate both descriptive and psychological aspects of the out-of-body experience, it also attempts to differentiate the prototype from other forms of altered mind/body perception. Hence, the book is useful for the clinician because it provides him or her with a thorough understanding of not only the out-of-body experience, but all states in which the mind/body relationship is perceived differently. These states form a continuum ranging from integrating and noetic experiences to highly pathological disturbances of body boundaries.

Out-of-body experiences and near-death experiences, in particular, have been subject to sensationalistic treatment by movies, popular books, and the media in general in recent years. One hears reports that proof of life after death has been provided by survivors of near-death experiences. Techniques of separating one's "soul" or one's "astral body" from one's physical body are advertised and taught. Another purpose of this book is to counterbalance such popularized treatments with an empirical examination of such states based on sound scientific rigor.

As psychiatrists and psychoanalysts, our frame of reference is primarily a psychoanalytic one. It is, however, a psychoanalytic viewpoint in broad dialogue with other disciplines, including philosophy, neurophysiology, religion, descriptive psychiatry, statistics, and parapsychology. We anticipate that purists of any persuasion, whether they be parapsychologists or orthodox psychiatric and psychoanalytic thinkers, will be critical of our approach to understanding these experiences. We hope that there is a substantial number of open-minded thinkers from all disciplines who will consider our ideas and our findings for what they are—a beginning effort to map uncharted waters with little more than a compass—and who will recognize that no single discipline can adequately address the complexity of these phenomena. We sincerely hope that more questions are raised than answers provided in the chapters that follow.

This tome represents the culmination of eight years of research. Our data base for this study of altered mind/body perception is a varied one. First, we draw on our questionnaire survey of 339 subjects who reported out-of-body experiences. This study represents the first large-scale, psychiatrically oriented research project designed to study persons who have reported out-of- body experiences. Our second source of data comes from intensive psychiatric and psychological evaluations of individual research subjects. Electroencephalographic studies of normal and "gifted" subjects constitute another portion of our data base. In addition our extensive psychoanalytic and psychotherapeutic work with subjects who have had experiences of altered mind/body perception provide rich clinical material that has furthered our understanding of these phenomena. Both of us have served as consultants at workshops devoted to the induction of altered states of consciousness, including states of altered mind/body perception; and our observations from these experiences have also contributed to our knowledge. Finally, we have drawn on the vast scientific literature from psychoanalysis, philosophy, parapsychology, and descriptive psychiatry, as well as from discussions with our colleagues, to build on what is already known about the phenomena we are studying.

We have divided our book into four sections. The first section defines and describes the out-of-body experience and reports the data from our questionnaire survey. The second section is devoted to the differentiation of the out-of-body experience from both pathological and normal states that may be confused with the experience. The third section focuses exclusively on the near-death experience. Our fourth and final section draws on concepts from psychoanalysis, from neurophysiology, from philosophy, and from religion to present an integrated view of how these experiences can be understood.

G.O.G.
S.W.T.

Part I
THE OUT-OF-BODY EXPERIENCE

One — A DESCRIPTIVE TYPOLOGY OF THE OUT-OF-BODY EXPERIENCE

Alterations in perception of the relationship between the mind and the body are of general interest to psychiatry, psychology, and philosophy for a wide variety of reasons. From our professional standpoint as psychiatrists and psychoanalysts, we are primarily interested in the psychology of these phenomena, whereas the parapsychologists often approach these experiences with the intent of determining whether something "really separates" from the body. Rogo (1984), a representative of this latter viewpoint, expresses the point of view that the out-of-body experience cannot be explained as simply a function of psychology. We do not share his view, which we believe implies an artificial separation between mind and body and places undue emphasis on provable separations. This "separationist" approach to the phenomenon reflects substantial philosophical and semantic problems, which we address in Chapter Thirteen.

DEFINITION

For the purposes of our questionnaire survey (Twemlow et al. 1982), which will serve as the primary focus of this chapter, we chose to define the out-of-body experience (OBE) in a very general way, since our review of the literature reveals that there is little, if any, agreement about what characterizes the state from the standpoints of phenomenology, physiology, or personality structure. For our questionnaire we chose the following definition: "An experience where you felt that your mind or awareness was separated from your physical body." We share Palmer's (1974) view that the only theme in the literature that distinguishes these experiences is a sense of location of the self at some place other than in the physical body. The definition of Broad (1966) is congruent with ours: "The experient has what appears to him at the time to be ordinary sense perceptions of actual things and persons (including very often his own physical body) from a point of view located in the ordinary space of nature outside the position occupied by his physical body at the time" (p. 167). We do not feel that it is wise to restrict our definition further at this point until the experience has been more thoroughly studied.

Such a definition, however, does reflect certain of our biases: 1) a belief that the subject is in a better position than the investigator to decide whether or not he or she has had an out-of-body experience; 2) a sense of location of self-awareness, rather than the complex and extremely variable visual and auditory experiences often reported in the anecdotal literature, is considered by us to be the core of the OBE; and 3) whether or not there is "objective" laboratory demonstration of the separation of self-awareness from its normal location in the head is irrelevant to the study of the phenomenon from a psychological point of view. The position of Osis (1973) that such a criterion should be fundamental to the experience is peripheral, in our view, to an understanding of its psychological impact on the individual, particularly in terms of his or her value system and the organization and functioning of his or her ego. The need to believe in the actual separation of consciousness from its normal location in the head will be considered further in Chapter Thirteen. Neurophysiological definitions of the phenomenon will be discussed in Chapter Twelve, although we recognize that these sorts of definitions cannot be said to characterize any phenomenon entirely adequately. There is, however, a modern bias toward the "objective truth" of laboratory measurements, so that such metaphors as the physiological accompaniments of subjective experience are viewed as having an unwarranted truthfulness and exactitude about them.

The term out-of-body experience was popularized by Tart, primarily to avoid the judgmental alternative names present in the parapsychological literature, which tend to imply exact knowledge of the etiology and nature of the experience. These names include such terms as astral projection, ESP projection, and astral travel. Some writers feel that the out-of-body experience is a specific form of psychopathology, a point that we will address in Chapters Three,

Four, and Five, while others, such as Ehrenwald (1974), place great emphasis on the visual perceptions of the self located "outside" of the body.

Tart's generally accepted definition of an altered state of consciousness is, "a qualitative alteration in the overall pattern of mental functioning, such that the experiencer feels his consciousness is radically different from the way it functions ordinarily" (1972). Using Tart's definition to build on our own, a complete definition of an out-of-body experience from these composite viewpoints might be: "an altered state of consciousness in which the subject feels that his mind or self-awareness is separated from his physical body and that this sense of self-awareness is more vivid and more real than a dream."

Semantic and definitional differences abound in OBE research, from our broad definition to Whiteman's (1956) much narrower and extremely detailed description of what an OBE should be. We perused the literature to see if the way in which the experience was defined altered the responses of the subjects studied. Blackmore (1982) surveyed Dutch and English students. One group of 98 students was given Palmer's (1979) OBE definition without further elaboration, while a matching group was provided with the same definition plus examples of OBEs, examples of lucid dreams, or with other information. She found no differences in the incidence of OBEs, with 18 percent of both populations reporting them. However, in a personal communication to us, she reported some design problems in her survey. Apparently, the Dutch translator made several errors, although Blackmore still asserts that the "only difference between groups was the amount of information they were given, not in the wording of the questions."

A TAXONOMY OF OBEs

These rather abstract definitions take on more life when they are fleshed out with actual reports of individual experiences. The examples we have gleaned from our research fall into several categories, which has allowed us to develop a rudimentary taxonomy or classification of OBEs. Our first example comes from one of approximately 700 letters we received describing such experiences. This report, which lacks many of the sensationalistic trappings of the experiences reported in the parapsychological and theosophical literature, is striking in its ordinary simplicity. Mr. A., a 53-year-old retired government employee, living in Puerto Rico, wrote of his experience as follows: "When I was approximately 10 years old, I was living together with my older brother at my uncle's house. One day, I was reclined on my bed, quite awake, and was looking at the ceiling beams of the old Spanish building where the living quarters were located. I was saying to myself many questions, such as what was I doing there and who was I. All of a sudden, I got up from the bed and started walking towards the next room. At that moment, I felt a strange sensation in me: it was a sensation of weightlessness and a strange mix of a sense of a feeling of joy. I turned back in my steps in order to go back to bed when to my big surprise, I saw myself reclined on the bed. This surprising experience at that very small age, gave me the kind of a jerk which, so to say, shook me back to my body."

This example exemplifies the ordinary, even mundane, content of the experience, its vivid emotional impact, the sense of a complete functioning self located outside the brain, and the considerable surprise when the physical body is seen. Also typical in this experience is the way the shock of seeing the body disrupts the delicate balance of the alteration of consciousness, causing a restitution of the normal cognitive set of the "in-body" state. Our example of this typical OBE does not resemble the dramatic anecdotal cases reported by gifted subjects such as Fox (1962), Muldoon and Carrington (1969), and Monroe (1977), the latter having reported over 580 personal OBEs. These experiences may be classified according to clustering patterns of certain descriptive features. The preceding typical example might be called the mundane type.

Another common type is analogous to mystical or religious experiences, as described by William James (1961). This form of OBE is particularly common when the subject is near death, as we will discuss in some detail in Chapters Seven, Eight, and Nine. This variety of OBE might well be termed the ecstatic type. The etymological origins of the word ecstasy imply that this form of out-of-body experience was well known in antiquity. Taken literally from the Greek roots of the word, ecstasy means "to stand outside of one's self," reflecting the ancient Greek people's awareness of the out-of-body phenomena associated with peak religious experiences. Out-of-body experiences tend to leave a deep imprint on the individual, very often with an ineffable, noetic quality. An experienced out-of-body subject, Mr. B., reported the following: "I laid down on the couch to rest, when I found myself being propelled upward by a tremendous force that was located between my shoulder blades. I found myself in a state of ecstasy, a state of great joy, and I was amazed by the power that was propelling me, as if it could move anything in the universe... I then became aware of the indescribably 'soft' substance that was smothering my face and found myself looking into and down a cable that appeared to be made of light itself. It was extraordinarily beautiful. Inside of it were untold trillions of tiny scintillating light fibers that also had a rolling motion like wind across a wheat field."

A third category illustrates the influence of a subject's belief system on the way in which the features of the experience are interpreted. We call this the esoteric type of out-of-body experience. These are primarily reported by those of a metaphysical bent and are generally conceptualized by the subjects as travels in the netherworld of "astral planes," where precognitive and mystical information is obtained. These individuals consider their travels to be "real" and the information valuable. They do not brook any questioning as to the authority of the information obtained from these esoteric out-of-body experiences. This category of OBE is much rarer, mainly reported by a small number of "gifted" subjects such as Robert Monroe (1977), who has described his encounters with alternative realities, complete with extraterrestrial-like entities and unknown civilizations. Monroe has reified his out-of-body experiences into a cosmology derived from information collected from these out-of-body travels over many years of exploration. In the esoteric form of out-of-body experience, the subject may view the OBE as an avenue into the discovery of cosmic truths.

Rarest of all is the nightmarish type of OBE. As we will demonstrate later in the chapter, the overwhelming majority of OBEs are pleasant. Occasionally, one encounters a frightening, nightmarish type of experience, which may or may not be a true OBE. For the sake of completeness, we provide an example here. A 34-year-old woman, Mrs. C., reported to us the following experience, which occurred when she was a 19-year-old college student. The event haunted her for the 15 subsequent years and eventually required therapeutic intervention. She describes it thusly: "I felt an invisible force pulling me strongly on my deep structures, the marrow of my bones came to mind. Its strength was such that eventually it lifted me horizontally into the air. I remember trying to feel with my hand as if I had actually left the bed. Always, at all moments, there was great pain, pressure, and terror. The pull of this force was strong, and I felt as if my heart would be ripped out of my chest. A great pressure was in my head, a rushing sensation and a sound similar to a vacuum cleaner. As it progressed, I would float horizontally in the bedroom, the blankets hanging from my body. Once I passed into the dormitory hall and tried to scream for help to a friend I saw there, but no sound would come. I headed for the bedroom window. I knew if I went out the window, I would die. I tried to resist the flow that was carrying me, once finding a pair of men's hands in midair to hang onto as an anchor. I passed through the concrete blocks of the bedroom wall and flew 15 to 30 feet away from the house."

HOW COMMON IS THE OUT-OF-BODY EXPERIENCE?

Individual case reports may make for interesting reading, but they tell us very little about the incidence of the experience in the general population. To explore this issue, we will turn away from anecdotes and look at the more scientifically rigorous surveys of large numbers of subjects. Early researchers tended to view the OBE as a rare phenomenon. These writers would seize on every individual report and analyze it in great detail based on metaphysical and theosophical assumptions (Myers 1903; Hill 1918; Muldoon and Carrington 1969; Fox 1962; and Yram 1965). These spontaneous cases were viewed as a direct window into the nature of the soul, the vindication of Cartesian mind/body dualism, and a gold mine of exciting information about the perennial problem of survival of bodily death. It is of interest historically that as psychical research developed in Britain and the United States, parapsychology in the United States, influenced by J.B. Rhine and his Duke University experiments, took a much more statistical and experimental bent. The British psychical research scene, on the other hand, remained highly metaphysical, eventually leading to a falling out between the two approaches (Mauskopf and McVaugh 1980).

Scientifically controlled surveys of the prevalence and incidence of out-of-body experiences are sparse. The first attempt was a pilot study by Hart (1954), conducted with Duke University sociology students in classes on operational sociology. Care was taken not to condition the students to psychical matters, but the method of sampling is called "representative" by Hart. No further information is available. Unfortunately, the study of 126 students was confounded by midstream alterations of the design. The students were initially asked if they had dreamed of standing outside of the body or floating in the air near the body, and this inquiry was later modified to a more complex definition involving having actually seen the physical body from a viewpoint completely outside of that body. Combining these two groups of 113 and 42 students, respectively, 27.1 percent of the 155 students reported having had an out-of-body experience, of which fewer than 8 percent said their OBEs had occurred only once. Green, of Great Britain, undertook two polls among Southampton college students and Oxford University students. She found that 19 percent and 34 percent, respectively, reported OBEs (Green 1967).

Besides these surveys of the incidence of out-of-body experiences in student populations, Green made a radio appeal in September 1966 for first-hand accounts of OBEs. She sent questionnaires to 400 persons who replied, and she received 326 responses to the first questionnaire and 251 to the second. The results of the survey are analyzed in detail in her book (Green 1968), where she reports that there is a definite predominance of women (68 percent) over men (32 percent), although her other studies of student populations show no significant sex differences.

The first random community mail survey of OBEs was conducted in 1974, using a random sample of 300 students at the University of Virginia and 700 adult residents of the Charlottesville, Virginia, area (Palmer 1979). A 46-item questionnaire was mailed to the subjects, inquiring about the incidence and characteristics of various psychic experiences. Information was also collected concerning attitudes toward the experience, the personal impact of the experience, and demographic data. Eighty-nine percent of the student sample and 51 percent of the town sample responded. Fourteen percent of the town sample and 25 percent of the students reported out-of-body experiences. Eighty-seven town subjects and 82 students reported more than one. Of those who had OBEs, 43 percent of the town subjects and 45 percent of the students saw their physical body, while 21 percent of the town respondents and 14 percent of the students reported traveling a distance from the physical body. Sixteen percent of the student subjects felt that they could produce out-of-body experiences at will, while only 12 percent of those from the town felt this way. The OBE subjects in the town sample tended to have significantly more vivid dreams, while in both the town and the student sample, there was a higher incidence of lucid dreams. The student sample reported more frequent mystical experiences. Personal dream analysis was commonly practiced among the subjects in the town sample. The OBE group in the town sample tended to use meditation more often than those who did not have OBEs.

Haraldsson (1977) found that 8 percent of 902 randomly surveyed adults, ages 30-70, in Iceland had first-hand familiarity with the out-of-body experience. In this well designed study, vigorous follow-up techniques were used, and an excellent 80 percent reponse rate was achieved, giving a highly representative sample of the adult population of Iceland. Psychic experiences in general were more common in women (70 percent), than in men (59 percent), with an overall high acceptance of psychic experience (66 percent).

Blackmore's (1984) random survey reported on 593 people selected from the electoral register for the city of Bristol, England. A return rate of 55.4 percent of useable questionnaires was obtained in her survey (12.2 percent) of 320 respondents who claimed to have had an out-of-body experience, with no significant age or sex differences between those with an OBE and those without one. Blackmore's survey used Palmer's broad defintion of the OBE, as did ours and Haraldsson's. Eighty-five percent of the subjects in Blackmore's survey had had more than one experience, but only 5 percent claimed to be able to produce it at will, a finding at variance with Palmer's survey. Blackmore (1978), in a nonrandom survey of 132 university students at Surrey, reported an OBE incidence of 11 percent under fairly stringent criteria. Students had attended lectures on the OBE and had been presented with a number of OBE case studies before participating in the survey. In 1975 and 1976 Kohr, using an identical instrument to Palmer's, surveyed nationwide members of the Association for Research and Enlightenment, a group of people interested in the writings of Edgar Cayce. This group has a national membership of approximately 20,000. Of the 400 respondents 50 percent claimed that they had had an out-of-body experience by Palmer's criteria, with 46 percent reporting one or two, and 26 percent, more than 9 such experiences. Significantly more females than males reported OBEs. This sample, of course, was highly biased. Irwin (1980) surveyed 177 students in an introductory psychology course at the University of New England in Australia. Thirty-six subjects (20 percent of the sample) reported an OBE within a broad definition similar to that used by our study and by Palmer. Using more stringent criteria, only 12 percent of the sample could be regarded as typical OBEs.

Myers et al. (1983), in a study of a student population, found that 23 percent of their 200 subjects had had OBEs, with 45 percent of those reporting at least one voluntary OBE. Only 36 percent saw their physical bodies, compared to 44 percent in Palmer's survey. About one-third of this sample had their OBEs in life-threatening circumstances. Age and sex were uncorrelated with OBE incidence or frequency, but significant correlations were found for use of mind-expanding drugs, practice of meditation, and mystical experiences.

Shiels, in 1978, conducted an anthropological survey of 67 non-Western cultures, 54 of which provided considerable detail about the incidence of beliefs in out-of-body experiences. Shiels' survey technique used the Human Relations Area Files (Murdock 1963), a group of coded files including microfilmed information on various cultures, all of which are ethnographically coded on a sentence-by-sentence basis, as the source. Sixty-seven cultures were examined. Detailed information was available on 54 cultures, indicating that OBEs are believed to occur in 95 percent of these cultures. They were absent in only 3 cultures—Apayao, U Islanders, and Platumans—that is, approximately 5 percent of the population. However, Mediterranean peoples were not well represented in these files, a potential source of bias in the sample. In 25 of the cultures (46 percent of the sample), the belief is that most or all people experience an OBE, while 23 cultures (43 percent of the sample) share the conviction that OBEs are experienced only by a minority of the population.

Shiels' study tests a theory proposed by Tylor in 1929, which suggested that the belief in the soul and in the out-of-body experience was based on dreaming. The idea was that if the sleeper spoke with a dead person during sleep, on awakening he or she might suppose that an immortal soul had survived physical death. In the 44 cultures for which adequate data were available, 14 saw all dreams as OBEs, and about a third did not see any dreams as OBEs. A number of other cultures felt that only especially gifted people, for example, shamans, could have an out-of-body experience. Over all, 31 percent distinguished between dreams that are OBEs and dreams that are merely dreams. Sheils concluded that Tylor's theory was not substantiated by the data of his survey.

Tart (1971) surveyed 150 experienced marijuana users (having used the drug more than 12 times) by circulating questionnaires on the University of California at Berkeley campus. He selected a population consisting of college students, their friends, and relatives. His percentage of subjects with a history of OBE—44 percent—compares well with the figures of Kohr (50 percent), whose sample was also skewed in a particular direction. Tart found that 23 percent of his subjects (34 users) had had one OBE, while 21 percent (32 users) had had multiple experiences. Slightly fewer males reported OBEs,

Table 1.1
QUESTIONNAIRE SURVEYS OF THE INCIDENCE OF OBEs

Source	Country	Sample	Method of Selection	Sample Size	%OBE
Hart (1954)	USA	College Students	Sociology class (no special emphasis on OBE)	155	27.1
Green (1967)	England	College Students	Undergraduate volunteers	115	19
Green (1967)	England	College Students	Student volunteers in ESP experiments	380	34
Tart (1971)	USA	Marijuana users on college campus	Experienced users (more than 12 times)	150	44
Haraldsson (1977)	Iceland	Adults Age 30–70 years	Random mail	902	11
Blackmore (1978)	England	College Students	Special lectures on OBE were given	132	11
Blackmore (1984)	England	City of Bristol Residents	Random mail	593	12.2
Palmer (1979)	USA	College Students	Random mail	268	25
		Charlottesville, VA Residents	Random mail	354	14
Irwin (1980)	Australia	College Students	Introductory psychology class (no special emphasis on OBE)	177	12
Kohr (1980)	USA	A.R.E. Members	Special interest group, mail survey	406	50
Myers (1983)	USA	College Students	Undergraduate psychology volunteers	200	23

but the males were more likely to have had multiple experiences. This trend is concordant with Green's results. Subjects who had had psychotherapy and/or a growth-promoting therapeutic experience tended to report more OBEs and more often reported multiple OBEs, as did users of stronger psychedelic drugs such as LSD. Although the OBEs reported were in conjunction with marijuana intoxication in 73 percent of the cases, it should be noted that 27 percent of Tart's subjects reported experiences while not smoking marijuana, thus confounding his figures. There were twice as many who considered that their OBEs began after they had started using marijuana, strongly suggesting that marijuana fosters the experience directly. Twice as many meditators, on the other hand, reported that their out-of-body experiences occurred before marijuana use. Similar proportions were present in the psychotherapy groups. Tart found that the experience is often interpreted as having "profound religious significance" (p. 106).

Osis (1979) surveyed 304 parapsychology teachers and other people with a vested interest in psychic phenomena about their OBEs. They typically reported rich and detailed visual experiences. Age and sex were evenly distributed, with 79 percent college educated and of nontraditional religious affiliations. Three-hundred-sixty-degree vision was often reported. Only 4 percent likened their experiences to dream imagery, and 86 percent stressed that OBEs were quite different from other ESP experiences. A high percentage claimed that fear of death was reduced and that their mental health improved over all, while 95 percent said that they would like to have another out-of-body experience. A summary of these surveys is contained in Table 1.1.

THE PHENOMENOLOGY OF THE OUT-OF-BODY EXPERIENCE

Our own questionnaire survey was designed to measure several dimensions of the out-of-body experience. We wanted to study the various preexisting conditions, the nature of the experience itself, and the impact of the experience on the subject. Another major area of interest to us was the psychological profile of the typical person who reports an out-of-body experience. Finally, we were interested in identifying demographic characteristics of the OBE subjects. Psychological and demographic data on our subjects will be discussed extensively in Chapter Two. Here we will confine ourselves to the preexisting conditions, the descriptive characteristics of the experience itself, and the impact on the experients. In describing our results, we are also defining the out-of-body experience as a phenomenological entity with characteristics that discriminate it from other experiences of altered mind/body perception. We will compare and contrast our data with that of other studies and conclude the chapter by delineating a prototype OBE, based on the salient features from our data.

Methodology

On February 15, 1976, one of us (S.W.T.), in an interview with a national periodical (circulation 15,000,000), solicited letters from people who thought they might have had an out-of-body experience. Of about 1,500 responses, 700 subjects reported experiences in which they felt their consciousness was separated from the physical body. About one year after the interview, two questionnaires (Profile of Out-of-Body Experiences, or POBE, and Profile of Adaptation to Life, or PAL) were sent to the 700 "positive" respondents. Of 420 people who returned valid questionnaires, 339 reported out-of-body experiences; 81 people did not have such experiences, but expressed a strong interest in learning about them and were used as a comparison group, controlling for high interest in esoteric phenomena.

The POBE is an anonymous multiscale questionnaire developed specifically for this study. Its design closely parallels that of the PAL, with a forced-choice format not exceeding four choices and space available for individual elaboration. The POBE explored possible preexisting conditions and phenomenological characteristics of the OBE by means of 51 items based on reports of near-death experiences, on mystical-religious literature, on philosophical-occult-psychic literature describing OBEs, and on psychoanalytic and psychiatric data describing depersonalization, psychotic, autoscopic, and hysterical states. Another 22 items questioned the range of possible feelings and reactions to the experience, both short-term and long-term. Five psychological test scales were included and are discussed in Chapter Two. Basic demographic data and the PAL questionnaire are also covered in Chapter Two.

Preexisting Conditions

Table 1.2 summarizes the conditions remembered to exist at the time that the out-of-body experience occurred. No cause-effect relationship can, of course, be definitively postulated between these

Table 1.2
PREEXISTING CONDITIONS

Attribute	Frequencies[1] Yes	No	%Yes
Physically Relaxed	263	70	79
Mentally Calm	261	69	79
Dreaming[2]	117	211	36
Meditating	88	241	27
Under Emotional Stress	74	250	23
Unusually Fatigued	51	279	15
Near Death	34	298	10
Experiencing Cardiac Arrest	17	313	5
Using a Drug	26	300	8
Under General Anesthesia	20	312	6
In Severe Pain	21	307	6
Experiencing Childbirth[3]	14	316	4
Involved in an Accident	13	318	4
Experiencing High Fever	11	320	3
Having a Sexual Orgasm	11	322	3
Drinking Alcohol	5	328	2
Driving a Vehicle	3	324	2

[1] Missing data account for discrepancies from the N of 339 valid responses received.
[2] In 97 Ss(83 percent), the dream was described as a "flying or falling" dream.
[3] 52.5 percent of sample were female, 178 respondents.

conditions and the experience itself, although such has been implied by some authors such as Crookall (1965). An overwhelming majority of our sample were in a relaxed and calm state of mind. Emotionally stressful conditions accounted for a much smaller percentage of our sample. The finding that this experience is not usually associated with illness or stress compares with similar findings by Crookall (1960). In his surveys 80 percent of his subjects were in a relaxed, normal state of mind at the time of the OBE. He even attempted to classify OBEs based on those occurring under physical and mental stress, and those occurring under nonstressful conditions. Green (1968), however, found that subjects who had had only one out-of-body experience were characteristically under some identifiable stress, usually physical trauma, prior to the experience.

Blackmore's random survey (1984) reports that 59 percent of OBEs occurred while resting or asleep, 31 percent while sleeping or dreaming, 26 percent during operations or accidents, and 18 percent while on drugs or medicines. In Shiels' (1978) cross-cultural survey, he found that of those cultures that believed in the occurrence of OBEs, sleep is believed to be the most common (80 percent) source of separation, with physical illness and emotional stress being less frequent but still important (75 percent). In many cultures, on the other hand, illness is thought to be a result, not a cause, of an out-of-body experience. The importance of a relaxed, nonpathological state as a preexisting condition for an OBE is prominent in his anthropological research, as well as in ours.

An impressionistic but scholarly paper surveying out-of-body experiences (Eastman 1962) asserts that they can occur in five different conditions: 1) dreaming, 2) just before and after sleep, 3) during hypnosis, 4) during serious illness, and 5) in drug states, including those induced by anesthetics and hallucinogens. Eastman also reports loneliness as a frequent emotion. Eastman's findings are similar to ours in the sense that she emphasizes a continuum of nonpathological states of relaxation proceeding to drowsiness.

Experimental attempts to induce an OBE have provided a laboratory perspective on preexisting conditions. Palmer and Vassar (1974) studied 60 voluntary subjects who attempted to induce an OBE through a progressive relaxation technique, audiovisual stimulation using random sounds, and rotating spiral disks, which were thought to facilitate the feeling of separateness from the body. The subjects would also voluntarily attempt to recreate a feeling of separation while imagining themselves traveling to another room. Forty-two percent of the subjects reported an OBE, and there were no meaningful correlations between the conditions and the proportion of subjects giving positive responses. Palmer found that "the experiences of the subjects were primarily proprioceptive and only about a third included distinct visual imagery" (p. 267).

The influence of belief systems as a preexisting condition for the OBE was tested by Smith and Irwin (1981), who found that a belief in immortality was not correlated with the incidence of out-of-body experience. In Green's (1968) sample, where one of every four of her cases were under purely psychological stress, the remainder were under a variety of physical stresses, including accidents and operations. She averred that chronic emotional stress or anxiety may produce several OBEs in a short period of time, whereas in other subjects, relaxed philosophical reflection, especially on existential questions, produces an out-of-body experience.

We subdivided our sample according to the total number of OBEs reported. Utilizing univariate independent group t-tests, we failed to find any precondition reaching the level of $p<.01$ for either the top 25 percent of the group or the bottom 25 percent. The latter group did, however, report significantly more spontaneous OBEs than the top 25 percent ($dF=62$, $p<.01$). We defined spontaneous OBEs as those which occurred without a volitional effort to leave the body. OBEs occurring during dreaming are distinguished emphatically by subjects as being "more real than a dream" in the vast majority of cases (94 percent). Flying and falling dreams comprise a majority of the dreams occurring at the time the OBE is noted. The certitude with which the subjects emphasized that they knew the difference between a dream state and an OBE state was impressive to us.

Subjects who were in a state of mental calmness at the time of the OBE had a significantly greater proportion of meditators ($dF=178$, $p<.001$) than the group of subjects who were not in such a state of mental calmness; otherwise, no other characteristics significantly differentiated these two groups.

There was a low incidence of drug and alcohol use in this population. The drugs that our subjects used were not classifiable, ranging from antihypertensives through vitamin pills and antibiotics. Only four subjects reported using psychedelic drugs (LSD and marijuana) at the time of the experience. These results contrast markedly with those of Tart (1971), in that our study suggests that drug intoxication is a relatively rare preexisting condition. Tart, however, surveyed quite a different population.

Seventy-four subjects provided individual descriptions of the types of emotional stress they were experiencing at the time of the OBE. Striking in these descriptions were the themes of loss, mourning, and loneliness, represented in 21 of the subjects. Threats of death, including illness, being in a war zone, presurgery, and cancer were present in 20, and marital and family problems in 12. When the descriptions were reviewed from the point of view of those who had only one OBE (n=33) versus those who had more than one (n=41), 21.7 percent of the one-OBE sample reported stress involving loss, mourning, and loneliness, compared with 34.2 percent of those who had more than one OBE.

A question was asked to explore why an individual might want to have an OBE. Of 91 classifiable responses, 19 (20.9 percent) were simply interested out of curiosity or for the simple purpose of having fun; 21 (21.3 percent) were members of a psychical research or study group; 23 (25.3 percent) were involved in personal, existential explorations associated with major developmental stages in their lives; and in 28 (30.7 percent) the experience was entirely spontaneous and unexpected. Only 10 percent of the sample had previously attended workshops on the subject of OBEs.

One final note on preexisting conditions is warranted regarding our subjects who reported that they were near death at the time of the OBE. Because of the popular literature on the subject of near-death experience, many people have the misconception that out-of-body experiences are most common when the subject is near death. Our study indicates that only 10 percent of persons who have out-of-body experiences are near death at the time of the OBE. This finding and its significance will be discussed at much greater length in Chapter Seven.

Nature of the Experience

Table 1.3 summarizes a number of phenomenological features of the experience itself. The first six features, which occurred in more than 50 percent of the subjects, do not illustrate the more esoteric aspects described in the literature. Rather, they detail a simple, subjective, perceptual experience of great vividness and reality. These characteristics suggest not only a sense of separation of the total self from its normal location in the head, but also an awareness that this self exists in the same environment as the physical body, which can be clearly seen. The OBE is typically associated with a feeling of unusual "energy" and a desire to return to the physical body.

As might be expected, some of the more vivid and detailed phenomenological features were overrepresented in the top 25 percent of the sample (that is, subjects who had had greater numbers of OBEs). Using group independent t-tests, the following features

Table 1.3
NATURE OF THE OUT-OF-BODY EXPERIENCE

Attribute	Frequencies[1] Yes	No	%Yes
Experience was more real than a dream.	315	19	94
Form of out-of-body figure similar to physical body.	232	73	76
OB figure in same environment as physical body.	197	123	62
Felt a sense of energy.	177	145	55
Wanted to return to body.	164	138	54
Felt able to pass through objects.	155	157	50
Felt vibrations in body.	128	204	38
Felt that part of awareness was still in body.	121	209	37
Was aware of presence of non-physical beings.[2]	120	203	37
Heard noises in early stages of the expericence.[3]	71	123	37
Experienced a change in time sense.	107	220	33
Saw a brilliant white light.[4]	96	225	30
Felt the presence of guides or helpers.	85	238	26
Experienced being in a dark tunnel with a white light at the end of it.	85	242	26
Felt attached to physical body.	68	259	21
Felt able to touch objects.	54	251	18
Felt that people not "out-of-body" were aware of presence.	45	277	14
Felt a sense of border or limit.	44	279	14
Experienced panoramic vision.	14	313	14

[1] Missing data account for discrepancies from the N of 339 total valid responses received.

[2] In 19 percent beings were people close to the subject, but whom had already died.

[3] A variety were reported, the most common being buzzing (29 percent), roaring (19 percent), music or singing (16 percent).

[4] 46 percent of this subsample (30) found the light strongly atrractive; 33 percent of the subsample felt it was a being trying to communicate with them.

were found to be more common in the top 25 percent: 1) a sense of energy (dF=94, p<.0005), 2) noises, particularly roaring noises (dF=39, p<.0005), 3) vibrations (dF=97, p<.01), 4) seeing the body from a distance (dF=97, p<.005), 5) a sense of being able to pass through objects (dF=93, p<.00006), 6) awareness of the presence of nonphysical beings (dF=96, p<.005), and 7) seeing a brilliant light (dF=96, p<.002).

Our findings show some similarities and differences from major studies reported in the literature. Hart (1954) analyzed cases that contained a veridical element. He examined 99 cases of what he termed "ESP projection." He found eight characteristics by a noncontrolled impressionistic clustering of cases. These were: 1) reported observation of distant places or persons through ESP; 2) an apparition was seen by the percipient during the experience; 3) the subject was aware of having been seen as an apparition; 4) the subject saw his or her own physical body during the experience from a spatially different viewpoint; 5) the subject saw himself or herself in a apparitional body; 6) this body defied gravity; 7) it passed through solid matter; and 8) it moved quickly through the air.

Crookall (1960, 1965) exhaustively performed nonveridical studies on the 746 first-hand accounts of out-of-body experience that he amassed. He found eight general characteristics, five of which corresponded to Hart's findings: 1) the subject viewed his or her own body from a spatially distinct vantage point; 2) he or she found himself or herself in an apparitional body; 3) this body was immune to gravity; 4) the perception might include ESP; 5) it might be seen as an apparition by a percipient; 6) the subject hovered above his or her physical body; 7) the physical and apparitional body were seen connected by a cord; 8) the percipient often saw forms representing discarnate beings during the experience. Crookall also emphasized the silver cord seen between the double and the body, which occurred in 20 percent of his "natural" (spontaneous and without stress) cases and 16.3 percent of his "enforced" (stress-induced) cases. Our study shows a 21 percent figure, close to his, whereas Green (1968) reports that only 3.5 percent of her 326 subjects reported seeing a physical connection such as a cord, although 29.6 percent of her subjects felt connected in some way to their physical bodies. Twenty-four percent of Blackmore's sample (1984) saw such a connection. Thus, it appears that Green's sample is unusual, while Crookall's anecdotal cases, our semirandom survey, and Blackmore's random survey are in closer agreement.

Seventy-six percent of our sample said that they seemed to be in a form similar to the physical body. Eighty percent of Green's subjects reported that they were a disembodied consciousness and were thus unaware of a substantial second or "astral" body during the experience. Blackmore's results were similar to ours; 69 percent of her subjects seemed to be in a complete body.

Green (1968) reports that 89 percent of her subjects felt that things appeared visually just the same as they ordinarily did, and 82 percent reported that objects were colored in the normal way. Only a minority of subjects described traveling to a landscape that did not resemble part of the world of normal experience. A small minority of her subjects described meeting with deceased relatives or other discarnate entities. Fifty-two percent of our sample described being in the same environment as the physical body, although 37 percent were aware of beings in nonphysical form. Vibrations and/or a sense of energy were present in only 12 percent of Blackmore's study, but in 38 percent of our subjects. A mere 8 percent of Blackmore's sample had the tunnel experience, with the presence of helpers or nonphysical beings present in just 5 percent of her cases. These figures were much higher in our sample.

Blackmore found that in 49 percent of the subjects, the experience was like dreaming, in striking contrast to our data, where 94 percent described the OBE as more real than a dream. Thirty-six percent of her subjects experienced the landscape as similar to the normal world, 24 percent said it was slightly vaguer, and only 15 percent compared it to a dream or fantasy. Only 44 percent of her subjects traveled away from their physical body. However, 56.5 percent of Green's radio-solicited sample actually claimed to have been more awake and more keenly observant than usual. She concludes that subjects usually find their intellectual faculties to be unimpaired during the OBE, often with a greater degree of clarity than usual.

In addition 89.3 percent of Green's sample felt that the experience seemed to be quite logical—not fantastic, although they also described it as "natural, complete, real, light, free, and full of vitality and health," in some respects an idealized state, not unlike the descriptive elaborations of our subjects. A variety of sounds were heard, varying from weird noises to choirs of angels singing. Ten percent of Blackmore's subjects heard "strange noises." Rogo (1975) attempts to classify OBEs by their music. He concludes that the Crookall "natural" type of experience tends to have more positive

Table 1.4
IMPACT OF THE OUT-OF-BODY EXPERIENCE

A.

During the Experience	Frequencies[1] Yes	No	%Yes
Calm, Peace, Quiet	281	90	72
Freedom	215	103	68
Sense of Purpose	182	115	63
Joy	173	139	55
No Special Feelings	91	161	36
Fear	111	209	35
Power	89	218	29
Sadness	39	267	13
Going Crazy	15	294	5
Immediately After the Experience			
Became Interested in Psychic Phenomena	266	46	85
Talked about it to Others	242	85	74
Curious	232	95	71
Felt Life Changed	188	127	60
Spiritual Experience	174	145	55
Felt he Possessed Psychic Abilities	136	180	43
Ordinary Event	120	195	38
Confused	87	233	27
Kept it Secret	77	237	25
Upset & Frightened	80	242	25
Forgot About It	20	295	6
Going Crazy	15	304	5

[1] Missing data account for discrepancies from the N of 339 total responses received.

B.

Longer Term Effect	Frequencies[1] Yes	No	%Yes
Like to Try Again	284	34	89
Developed Greater Awareness of Reality	281	47	86
Very Pleasant	273	47	85
Lasting Benefit	240	67	78
Change Towards a Belief in Life After Death	215	109	66
Great Beauty	208	112	65
Like Travelling to Far Off Land	165	149	53
The Greatest Thing that Ever Happened	136	177	43
Reminiscent of Childhood Experiences	68	248	22
Disappointing	20	299	6
Like Being Drunk or High	20	297	6
Mentally Harmful	7	313	2

[1] Missing data account for discrepancies from the N of 339 total responses received.

music, and the Crookall "enforced" OBEs, including anesthesia, drowning, and suffocation, as well as deliberate projections, typically have less positive qualities to the music. Green (1968) does not emphasize the phenomenon of noises at all. In our subjects 37 percent did hear noises, but there was no natural division as suggested by Rogo and Crookall. For example music or pleasant sounds accounted for only 16 percent of the sample. However, the vast majority of our sample would fall under Crookall's "natural" category.

Impact of the Experience

Table 1.4 summarizes the reactions of the subjects to the out-of-body experience. A majority of our respondents had remarkably positive experiences. The use of superlative adjectives in the reports is striking. As would be expected, *t*-tests revealed that those subjects who were in a state of mental calmness at the time of the OBE experienced more positive affects both during and after the experience. Affective states such as joy (dF=304, p<.01), freedom (dF=309, p<.008), and calm, peace, and quiet (dF=90, p<.0002) were experienced much more frequently than in those who had feelings of fear during the experience. In addition t-test comparisons also revealed the fact that those who were mentally calm had more detailed and vivid experiences than those who experienced fear at the time of the OBE. For example they were more likely to have a sense of energy (dF=312, p<.02), to hear vibrations (dF=332, p<.01), and to feel that people not "out-of-the-body" were aware of their presence (dF=155, p<.008).

In the mentally calm group, the experience was seen as having a more lasting and dramatic impact on their lives. For example it was described as a spiritual or religious experience (dF=302, p .01), an experience of great beauty and lasting benefit (dF=301, p .0003), and it was said to have effected a change toward a belief in survival after death (dF=331, p .01). One possible explanation for these differences is that those persons who experienced fear were actually experiencing depersonalization or nightmares, as we shall discuss further in Chapters Three and Six, respectively.

Subjects who described a sense of purpose to the experience, indicated that it enabled them to obtain closure on some of the major existential questions of their lives. These accounts reflect a preponderance of subjects who were dealing with issues associated with major life changes and requiring much introspection, review, and assessment of personal strengths and weaknesses.

On the issue of impact, there is much agreement among studies. Almost never is the out-of-body experience considered to be trivial in its impact by the subjects, even if the actual experience itself contains nothing particularly startling. Blackmore's random sample, in fact, had the fewest number of people who really enjoyed the experience. Only 10 percent claimed that it had changed their lives, compared with more than half the respondents in our study. A majority of Green's subjects described the experience positively, if not ecstatically. Twenty-eight percent of Blackmore's subjects found the experience frightening, and only 28 percent enjoyed the experience. Blackmore's study is quite unusual in this regard. Her randomized design is more likely to pick up subjects who did not enjoy the experience than the self-selected methodology of our survey and those of others, where the subjects may well respond because they enjoyed the OBE and wish to discuss it. Our study is similar to Crookall's, Green's, and Osis'. Crookall found that 14.5 percent of his "natural" category had a paradiselike experience and only 1.8 percent, an experience similar to descriptions of hell.

The metapsychological significance of the experience will be further explored in Chapter Ten. What is obvious, however, is that the responses are quite reminiscent of categories used to describe peak experiences (Maslow 1970) and mystical religious conversions (James 1961). However, the ambivalent effect often described in mystical experience appears not to be so prominent here. Our subjects emphasize the heightened clarity and vividness of the real world, as well as an increasing sense of its logical coherence, an increased feeling of harmony, and a sensation of being integrated with the real world. The experience appears to stimulate the individual to explore the world of parapsychology and esoteric phenomena. The individual typically develops an increased sense of uniqueness and autonomy and begins an inner search for ways in which meaning can be assigned to this extraordinary experience that seems to transcend the ordinary paradigms of reality as we know it.

CONCLUSION

Our questionnaire study has a variety of defects in addition to those usually associated with questionnaires. For example the experiences are remembered often from many years before, and the questionnaire is in forced-choice directive form. However, a large number of questions were asked. Even though individualized protocols were not used, the generalizability of the data is aided by the semi random nature of the study and the anonymity of the respondents. It should be noted that the profile of respondents to this questionnaire is different from a profile of typical respondents to the news magazine used. Consultation with the editors of the magazine indicated that they considered their typical readership to be a 20-25-year-old housewife and mother of two small children, who spends several hours each day watching television. Actually the study population turned out to be highly representative of the general population at large.

Although in 30 percent of our subjects, a vegetative form of consciousness remained within the body, the sense of the whole self is located somewhere other than in its usual place in the brain, even in that group. Both observing and experiencing ego functions are located at a point in perceptual space other than the brain, with the physical body being seen as inert and thoughtless. Consciousness is not clouded in the vast majority of cases, and the perception of the subjects that the OBE is far more real than a dream is clear. Subjects who are fearful during the OBE tend to have a more negative reaction, as might be expected, and tend to utilize the experience for much less attitudinal change, with the experience remaining much less vivid in their memories. Such experiences may well be examples of depersonalization or other psychopathological disturbances that we will consider in detail in Chapters Three, Four, and Five.

The data of our questionnaire survey allow us to delineate a prototypical OBE, with full awareness that such a composite experience only describes the majority of experiences and that many variations exist. This typical experience occurs in a state of physical relaxation and mental calmness. Emotional stress is usually absent. The experience itself is quite pleasant, and the subject typically feels sensations of calm, peace, and quiet during the OBE. He or she may even experience joy. Unpleasant affects are much less common. A feeling of going crazy is quite rare. The subject is likely to find himself in the same environment as his or her physical body, which he or she sees in an inert state below his or her point of perception, which is spatially separate from his or her physical body. The subject also notes that he or she has a "new body" in a form asimilar to his or her physical body. The experience itself is vivid in quality and clearly more real than a dream state. The OBE typically has a profound influence on the individual's subsequent life. The subject is likely to feel that his or her life was changed by the experience. The subject may well view it as a spiritual experience and is likely to believe in life after death as a result of the OBE. The individual has a certain fascination about the experience and probably would like to try it again. He or she may even feel that it is one of the greatest events of his or her life.

Two — A PSYCHOLOGICAL AND DEMOGRAPHIC PROFILE OF PERSONS REPORTING OUT-OF-BODY EXPERIENCES

Our review of the psychiatric and parapsychological literature found very few studies that include detailed psychological profiles of people who claim to have out-of-body experiences. In our questionnaire study (Jones et al. 1984) we attempted to remedy this lack of information by asking the following questions:

1. Will subjects who report out-of-body experiences be more prone to imaging and fantasy?
2. Will subjects who have OBEs have lower anxiety about death?
3. Will more hysteroid responses be found in subjects who have OBEs?
4. Will there be more indication of psychoticism among subjects who claim such experiences?
5. Will people who have OBEs tend to be danger-seeking?
6. Are persons reporting out-of-body experiences psychiatrically disturbed or psychologically well-adjusted?
7. What are the demographic characteristics of people who have OBEs?

These questions are relevant, as Walsh (1980) has observed, because of the tendency for clinicians to "pathologize" their interpretations of various states of altered consciousness. For example, out-of-body and dissociative types of experiences have been reported as typical symptoms in patients suffering from hysterical and psychotic disorders (DSM III 1980). It is not uncommon for people who have such experiences to be diagnosed as suffering from some form of psychiatric illness. Kennedy (1976), for example, writes of out-of-body experiences in a paper entitled, "Self-induced Depersonalization Syndrome." He reports two cases of "ego-syntonic depersonalization," both of which appear to be out-of-body experiences. The term "ego-syntonic depersonalization" is a contradiction in terms, since by definition, depersonalization is ego-dystonic, as we will elaborate in Chapter Three. The danger-seeking scale was included because a review of the parapsychological and theosophical literature found covert or overt emphasis on the great value of courageously traveling the "astral planes" and seeking contact with unknown realms to improve the fund of human knowledge.

INSTRUMENTS

In addition to the phenomenological questions discussed in Chapter One, our POBE questionnaire contained a series of psychological scales used to assess whether or not persons who had OBEs had any discriminating psychological features. The choice of scales was dictated by the research questions stated previously. Scale I is *Attitudes to Imaging and Fantasy* and contains the 37 items of the "Absorption" scale extracted from Tellegen's *Differential Personality Questionnaire* (DPQ) (1974). Also, from this questionnaire are nine "danger-seeking" items, which are similar to "stimulus-seeking" scale items. The DPQ is a factor-analytically derived instrument that was standardized on a normal population. The "Absorption" scale is a measure of the capacity for episodes of absorbed and "self-altering" attention that are sustained by imaginative representations. Individuals become absorbed with "a full commitment of available perceptual, motoric, imaginative, and ideational resources to a unified representation of the attentional object." Scale II is *Attitude to Self and Others* and includes the *Hysteroid Scale* developed by Caine (1972), which is derived from a scale that measures both obsessoid and hysteroid attitudes and cognitive styles. Also contained here are the 20 items of Eysenck's *Psychoticism Scale* (1968). Scale III, *Attitudes Toward Death*, is represented by ten items of the *Death Anxiety Scale* of Dickstein (1972). These ten items are those that we have found discriminate best between high and low death anxiety.

Profiles of Adaptation to Life (PAL)

This questionnaire is one of the very few that is designed to assess the mental health of populations who are not necessarily identified as patients and who have not had circumscribed treatment experiences (Ellsworth 1981). Thus, the scale is ideally suited for our population.

A sample of 1,738 subjects was used to establish reliability and validity of the PAL scale using the 154-item research form. Six-hundred-and-seventy-eight subjects were patients from two states seeking psychiatric care but who were not, at the time of the study, in treatment. One hundred and twenty-one subjects were people who had been selected for training in Transcendental Meditation (TM) but had not yet been trained. They came from California, Massachusetts, New York, and Virginia. Ninety-six of the subjects were students, mostly in nursing and psychology, in a community college. Four-hundred-and-thirty-five subjects were respondents to our OBE studies (only 420 of them provided adequate information for inclusion in the study reported in Chapter One). Three-hundred-and-sixty-six were people enrolled in the M-5000, an altered states of consciousness program conducted by Robert Monroe, which has as one of its goals the inducement of an out-of-body experience. Forty-two participants were mental health professionals invited to a conference on altered states of consciousness and represented those largely on the forefront of research in this area.

The PAL scale measures seven areas of adjustment:

1. *Negative emotions.* This factor is composed of items that measure feelings described as "uneasy, troubled, gloomy, tense, unhappy and worried." A number of items were derived from the existing *Profile of Moods Scale* (1971), and these reflect the consensually held viewpoint that the absence of such symptoms as anxiety and depression represents good adjustment.

2. *Psychological well-being.* This item measures whether or not one enjoys talking with others, whether one finds work interesting, and whether one feels trusting, involved, needed, and useful. It is basically a dimension that measures positive adjustment to life. It reflects the extent to which people are experiencing a sense of self-worth and enjoyment in their lives.

3. *Income management.* This item focuses on how well people handle the money available to them, including feeling free from

worry about debts, having enough money to pay bills, and handling unexpected expenses.

4. *Physical symptoms.* This factor measures the reported frequency of headaches, fever, dizziness, nausea, and the use of prescribed or over-the-counter remedies for headaches and stomach problems. Such items are often considered to be "psychosomatic," implying a relationship between emotional and physical health. It is also a measure of illness-consciousness or the extent to which people focus on physical problems (hypochondriasis).

5. *Alcohol and drug abuse.* This item measures the frequency of drug and alcohol use and whether there are family and cognitive problems associated with the abuse.

6. *Close interpersonal and child interpersonal relationships.* In this dimension, if the person lives with another adult, a spouse or parent, he or she is asked to indicate the quality of that relationship by answering questions describing the extent to which they talk over angry feelings, spend enjoyable time together, discuss important matters, feel close, and agree on friends. If the person lives where there are children in the home, the quality of that relationship is measured by such questions as time spent talking to children, feelings of closeness, doing things together, and treating each other with respect.

The strength of the PAL scale is that it focuses on actual behavior rather than on the reported subjective mood states, a defect of many of the psychiatrically oriented scales.

MENTAL HEALTH OF OBE SUBJECTS

Table 2.1 gives comparative factor scores for the six groups to whom the research form of the PAL scale was administered. The OBE group is significantly freer from negative emotions than clinic patients, TM trainees, or college students, but not significantly different from M-5000 trainees and professionals. While the professional group had the highest sense of psychological well-being, the OBE group is also significantly higher in psychological well-being than clinic patients and TM trainees. Income management is most difficult for the clinic clients, who are significantly poorer in this area than the OBE group and all other groups. The OBE group had significantly fewer psychosomatic symptoms as well, strikingly different from the clinic patients and TM trainees, who were significantly higher in

Table 2.1
PAL SCORES FOR DIFFERENT GROUPS USING ANOVA

	Clinic Clients	TM Trainees	Community College Students	OBE	M-5000[2] Trainees	Professionals	F Ratio
A. Negative Emotions	16.89[1]	14.31[1]	12.80[1]	11.13	10.69	10.50	236*
B. Psychological Well-Being	11.26[1]	13.12[1]	15.56	15.44	16.25	17.52[1]	136*
C. Income Management	7.85[1]	8.86	9.16	9.26	9.72	9.65	53*
D. Physical Symptoms	13.57[1]	11.50	10.94	9.77[1]	9.21	8.67	147*
E. Alcohol-Drug Abuse	6.45[1]	7.02[1]	5.64	5.50	6.00	5.62	14*
F. Close Relations	10.74[1]	13.97	14.48	14.55	15.74	16.74	67*
G. Child Relations	13.69	13.91	14.36	15.64	15.69	15.38	11*

* $p < .001$ for 5 by 1703 dF.

[1] Group mean is significantly different from all other groups.

[2] An altered states of consciousness training program developed by Robert Monroe, author of *Journeys Out of the Body*, Garden City, NY: Anchor Doubleday, 1977.

alcohol and drug use than all other groups. The OBE group, when comparing the means, had the lowest value of all groups for the alcohol and drug use factor. As expected, close adult interpersonal relationships were poorest in the clinic patients. There were no significant differences between groups in child interpersonal relationships.

Overall, the OBE group represents a very close approximation of the "average healthy American." They were significantly healthier in a psychological sense than the clinic patients and TM trainees, who tended to be the poorest in adjustment. They were also significantly better adjusted than a randomly selected group of college students. On the average there were few significant differences between the OBE group and the two professional groups—the M-5000 program and the professional conference attendees.

To determine if there were any significant differences between the OBE subjects and the non-OBE comparison group on the psychological test scales, we compared the means of the two groups using two-tailed univariate independent group tests. No significant differences were found on the scales measuring death anxiety, psychoticism, hysteria, and "absorption." The *Danger-Seeking Scale* was an exception. On these nine items, the non-OBE group's mean was significantly higher ($t=2.0013$, $df=418$, $p<.05$) than the OBE group, indicating that those persons who had the OBEs were less danger-seeking than those who had an interest in the experience but had not actually had an OBE. As Quay (1965) points out, a number of people with a variety of psychiatric disorders, including psychopathic personalities, wish to increase rather than decrease stimulation. Such increases in stimulation may be pleasurable.

Hence, we found that the OBE group was significantly healthier than a variety of other normative groups in the population and did not have the constellation of symptoms often equated with character disorders, such as psychosomatic disorders, alcohol and drug abuse, or stimulus seeking.

Irwin (1980), in a small study of 21 Australian undergraduates, found large differences in the "Absorption" scale between OBE subjects and controls, with the former tending to be more internally absorbed. He also concluded that OBE subjects were not disposed to be either verbalizers or visualizers, and were "rather neurotic." In another, even smaller study ($n=13$) (1981), he found that the OBE group tended to exhibit a lower need for achievement on the *Edwards Personal Preference Scale*. The generalizability of Irwin's results is, of course, limited by the very small size of his sample. In a slightly larger substudy of 34 subjects who had had near-death experiences (Twemlow and Gabbard, in press), we found significantly higher "Absorption" scores in the near-death as compared with the OBE group, a finding that deserves further research. Also, as discussed in Chapter Six, OBE dream subjects had significantly higher "Absorption" scores as compared to other OBE subjects.

Myers et al. (1983) report a small study of 45 OBE subjects who were undergraduate Catholic college psychology students. These subjects showed significantly higher "Absorption" scores and internal-locus-of-control scores than a peer control group. They also found their subjects to have a higher score on imaginative fantasy activity. No significant differences were found for death anxiety or for religiosity, confirming our results and those of other studies.

Research to determine whether or not it is possible for healthy individuals to have experiences of this type is in its infancy. An interesting study of the personality correlates of mystical experience (Hood et al. 1979) attempted to delineate stable personality correlates of mystical experience using a health-oriented personality instrument, the *Jackson Personality Inventory*. The OBE has many characteristics of the mystical experience, especially in its life-changing effect on the individual. Hood found that the person reporting a mystical experience may be described as "one with a breadth of interests, creative and innovative, tolerant of others, socially adept and unwilling to accept simple solutions to problems. This person is likely to be highly critical of tradition." Hood's work implies that one can have mystical experiences without being psychiatrically disturbed.

Myers et al. (1983) also used the *Jackson Personality Inventory* with their OBE subjects. Supporting Hood's findings for mystical experience in general, they describe the typical OBE subject as having "high levels of breadth of interest and innovativeness. These subjects also see themselves as responsible, honest, and stable, as well as curious, intellectual, analytical and sociable, although low in conformity and value orthodoxy" (p. 142).

Our results, while showing no evidence of psychiatric illness in our population, do not lead us to commit the logical fallacy of interpreting positive findings from negative results. We simply leave the findings of this large-scale study as a stimulus for future research. We will, however, point out two conclusions that the study did demonstrate: 1) there was not measurable psychopathology in the OBE group; and 2) the OBEers did demonstrate considerably higher levels of health than many other groups in the population, who were not identified patients, such as college students and TM trainees. In some respects the OBEers were healthier than the M-5000 trainees and approximated the health of the highly educated research conference attenders. Thus, the OBE group actually seems to be psychologically remarkably healthy rather than simply lacking in illness.

DEMOGRAPHIC VARIABLES

Table 2.2 lists the demographic profile of the PAL groups. Of the OBE respondents 47.5 percent were male and 52.5 percent were female. The ages ranged from 12 to 83 with a mean age of 44.6 years.

Table 2.2
DEMOGRAPHIC PROFILE OF PAL GROUPS

	Clinic Clients	TM Trainees	Community College Students	OBE Ss	Non-OBE Ss	M-5000 Trainees	Professionals
Marital Status							
Married	46	34	34	51	51	49	64
Widowed, Separated, or Divorced	35	16	10	27	25	30	17
Single	19	50	56	31	23	21	17
Sex							
Male	26	47	21	47.5	50	52	86
Female	74	53	79	52.5	50	48	14
Education							
Less than High School	29	13	0	18	25	1	0
High School Graduate	37	27	0	27	15	6	0
Some College	22	34	97	35	24	38	7
College Graduate	12	26	3	20 / 6*	36 / 14*	54	93
Age							
Mean Age in Years	30.2	28.0	24.4	44.6	44.4	39.2	41.4
Under 21	15	39	53	8	7	16	13
21-40	71	45	45	36	36	52	49
41-60	13	13	2	41	41	31	36
61 and Over	1	3	0	15	16	1	2
Income Source							
Work	47	57	46	51	55	68	90
Spouse Relative or Friend	36	35	40	22	20	20	5
Other	17	8	14	27	25	12	5

* Advanced degrees

Note: numbers express percentages.

Fifty-one percent were married, 23 percent single, and 25 percent separated, widowed, or divorced. The subjects lived in 38 states and three foreign countries. Educationally, the OBE group exceeds that of the U.S. population as determined in the 1970 census, where "less than high school" accounted for 34 percent of the population, "high school graduate" for 36 percent of the population, "some college" 14 percent of the population, and "college graduate" for 16 percent of the population (U.S. Statistical Abstracts 1978). Osis (1979) reports that 79 percent of his sample of 304 subjects attended college, compared to 55 percent of our sample.

Table 2.3 lists the occupational profile. A wide range of occupations was represented in the sample, varying from unemployed individuals to physicians and other doctoral level professionals. Of the occupational groups listed, the most striking differences between OBE and non-OBE subjects are found in the group of housewives, where 19.84 percent of the OBE subjects were represented versus 9.84 percent of the non-OBE subjects; students, where 7.8 percent of the OBE subjects were found as opposed to 14.7 percent of the non-OBE subjects; and the professional group, in which 16.7 percent of the OBE subjects were represented compared to 22.1 percent of the non-OBE subjects.

Our results concerning sex differences in OBE are in striking contrast to those of Green (1968). She found in her survey of 326 OBE subjects that 68 percent of her subjects were women, while only 32 percent were men. Our sex distribution, on the other hand, was approximately even, while our age range was highly variable, as were Osis' (1979) and Green's (1968) populations. Green (1967), in another survey of university students, found no significant difference between OBE incidence in males and females, nor any differences between science and art students, between scholars and "commoners," or between those educated in public versus private schools.

In Palmer's (1979) community mail survey of psychic experience, the separated and divorced subjects had a relatively high incidence of out-of-body experiences, 35 percent in the former and 13 percent in the latter, a statistically significant difference at $p<.05$. There were no other significant differences in Palmer's survey for age, sex, race, birth order, politics, religion, education, occupation, or income category for the out-of-body experience subjects as compared with the other non-OBE questionnaire participants. Blackmore (1984) also found no significant age or sex difference between OBE and non-OBE subjects in her random survey. In a recently published

Table 2.3
OCCUPATIONAL PROFILE

Occupation	OBE %	OBE Frequency	Non-OBE %	Non-OBE Frequency
Business, Professional Administrative	16.74	54	22.14	18
Technician	8.68	28	4.92	4
Clerical	6.20	20	7.38	6
Sales	4.65	15	4.72	4
Self-Employed Artists, Writers, Musicians	6.51	21	3.69	3
Manually Skilled Laborers	8.06	26	9.84	8
Semi-Skilled Laborers	4.64	16	9.84	8
Unskilled Laborers	2.48	8	3.69	3
Housewives	19.84	64	9.84	8
Student	7.75	25	14.26	12
Unemployed	4.24	14	2.46	2
Retired	9.67	21	6.15	5
Other	1.24	4	0	0

Total Frequency: OBE = 322
Non-OBE = 81

Italian survey (Giovetti 1983), two-thirds of 110 OBE subjects were men, with a random spread of age, education, and sociocultural level.

The religious background of the respondents, as well as their current religion, is listed in Table 2.4. In the OBE group only 51 percent were still associated with the same religion as before their out-of-body experience, whereas among the subjects who did not have an OBE, 61 percent are currently affiliated with the same religion as they identified under "religious background." Similarly, Osis (1979) found: "religious affiliations were somewhat biased toward the nontraditional groups" (p. 51). However, while this is a trend in our data, the difference is not statistically significant. In order to look at the possible effects that the number of OBEs have on current religious preference, the subjects who had one out-of-body experience were contrasted with those who had multiple experi-

Table 2.4
RELIGION

A. Subjects With OBE

Religious Background		Current Religion	
Roman Catholic	28%	Roman Catholic	14%
Protestant	53%	Protestant	30%
Jewish	1%	Jewish	0%
Other	11%	Other	30%
None	6%	None	26%

B. Subjects Without OBE

Religious Background		Current Religion	
Roman Catholic	32%	Roman Catholic	22%
Protestant	56%	Protestant	30%
Jewish	0%	Jewish	0%
Other	5%	Other	24%
None	7%	None	24%

ences. Fifty-seven percent of the subjects who reported one out-of-body experience remained with their background religion. By contrast, among those who had multiple OBEs, only 46 percent remained with their original religion. Again, a trend is noted, but the difference is not statistically significant.

Interpretation of the out-of-body experience differed according to religious affiliation. Those subjects who professed a current religious affiliation were more likely than the nonaffiliated group to view their out-of-body experience as being of a religious or spiritual nature as determined by two-tailed univariate independent group t-tests (df=309, p<.0001). Similarly, the religiously affiliated group were also likely to interpret the OBE as evidence that they had special psychic abilities (df=307, p<.001). Finally, the religiously affiliated group also felt that there was a purpose to their OBE significantly more often than the nonaffiliated group (df=299, p<.008).

OBEs have been connected with religious and mystical literature for many centuries. The connection between religious and meditative

Table 2.5
EXPERIENCE WITH ALTERED STATES OF CONSCIOUSNESS
(drug-induced and not drug-induced)

For OBE Subjects Only

Marijuana or Hashish—(check one)	
☐ Never	75
☐ Former user (not for a year)	7
☐ Infrequent use (once a month or less)	10
☐ Occasional use (2 to 3 times a month)	3
☐ Frequent (at least once a week, but not every day)	4
☐ Heavy use (every day)	2
Psychedelics— (e.g., LSD, check one)	
☐ Never	89
☐ Less than three times	5
☐ 3-25 times	5
☐ More than 25 times	1
Other Non-Prescription Drugs (check any number)	
☐ None	51
☐ Narcotics (heroin, morphine, cocaine)	5
☐ Amphetamines (speed)	10
☐ Alcohol	39
☐ Tranquilizers (e.g., Valium, barbiturates)	16
Have you ever been hypnotized or practiced Self-Hypnosis?— (check one)	
☐ Never tried	48
☐ Tried but wasn't able to be hypnotized	21
☐ Less than three times	9
☐ 4-12 times	6
☐ More than 12 times	21
Have you read literature or attended presentations and workshops in the following areas in the past year? (check any number)	
☐ Drug use and abuse	12
☐ Meditation and spiritual disciplines	51
☐ Hypnosis	25
How often have you Meditated in the last month? (check one)	
☐ Not at all	38
☐ Once daily	16
☐ More than once a day	11
☐ 1-3 times per week	13
☐ Occasionally when I think of it	22

If you practice Meditation, please check the following.

I use mainly:
☐ Transcendental Meditation 14
☐ Other type (e.g., Kundalini) 16
☐ My own type (not from any special discipline) 61
☐ No answer 9

Note: Numbers express percentages.

practices in our study is far from clear, however. Although there appears to be a diminished interest in traditional religions in our subjects, certainly no cause-effect relationship can be asserted between this drop-off in religious interest and the out-of-body experience. What is clear is that those persons who consider themselves religious are much more likely to interpret the out-of-body experience as part of their personal religious system. In this regard the experience might be compared with that of the religious conversion experience.

Experience with a variety of altered states of consciousness, drug-induced and not drug-induced, are listed in Table 2.5. Drug usage was comparable to average figures for the adult U.S. population. For example, 75 percent of the population had never used marijuana. Eighty-nine percent had never used psychedelic drugs, and 51 percent reported never using any of the other categories of drugs.

People with little or no experience with hypnosis were compared with those who had been hypnotized or had used self-hypnosis more than 12 times (Table 2.5). The experienced hypnotic group, who were presumably used to consciousness-alteration techniques, were significantly less frightened during the experience compared with groups who were not experienced with hypnosis ($df=138$, $p<.003$). Forty-four percent of the population had never been hypnotized while 12 percent had been hypnotized more than 12 times.

Although our study did not show a higher absorption score in the OBE group, Irwin's (1980) data did. Tellegen (1974) has regarded absorption as a personality trait closely related to susceptibility to hypnosis. The literature has attempted to connect out-of-body experiences and hypnotic susceptibility (Palmer and Lieberman 1976; Wilson and Barber 1982). Wilson and Barber (1982) studied 27 excellent and 25 poor hypnotic subjects. Eighty-eight percent in the excellent group reported OBEs, compared to only 8 percent in the poor subject group. Our group certainly had a high percentage of people who had been exposed to hypnosis. However, there were no significant differences when the OBE and non-OBE populations were compared.

Meditation questions were included on the questionnaire because of the reports in the literature of an association between OBEs and meditation (Maliszewski et al. 1981). Sixty-two percent of the OBE respondents described themselves as meditating at frequencies varying from once daily to "occasionally, when I think of it," and for an average of nearly nine years. Of this group 61 percent used idiosyncratic techniques including simple introspection, daydreaming, and prayer. Obviously, this wide definition of meditation resulted in an artificially inflated figure. A similar percentage (63 percent) of subjects in the comparison group described themselves as meditators. Two-tailed univariate independent group t-tests indicated that meditators were more likely to have experienced the OBE as joyful ($df=294$, $p<.003$) and peaceful ($df=288$, $p<.002$) as compared to nonmeditators. Although meditation has been anecedotally linked to the occurrence of out-of-body experiences, this association has not been substantiated in our study, as both the OBE group and the non-OBE group contain similar percentages of meditators.

Our exploration of the psychological and demographic characteristics of persons who have had out-of-body experiences is only a beginning effort. More extensive study with more finely tuned instruments will be required to define accurately individual characteristics of persons whose consciousness is altered in this way. However, our studies would seem to indicate that it is premature and unfounded to categorize out-of-body experiences as always delusional, illusionary, or drug-induced.

At the end of Chapter One, we summarized our data in the form of an OBE prototype. If we attempt to summarize the material from this chapter in a similar manner, the "typical profile" of the OBE subject is remarkably similar to the average, healthy American individual. The individual may be of any age and is equally likely to be male or female. If an adult, he or she is likely married and probably has attended college. This individual works regularly at any of a number of jobs. If he or she is actively religious, the OBE will be seen as spiritually important. Our prototypical subject might practice a nontraditional religion, if religious at all, and may have a history of changing from traditional to nontraditional religion after the OBE. His or her psychological health is generally excellent, ranking with the healthiest groups in the population, notably in certain areas, such as in the absence of alcohol and drug abuse. He or she has no sign of psychotic thinking, nor is there any indication of hysterical tendencies. Our typical OBE subject tends to be less of a thrill seeker than many others around him or her, and he or she lacks any of the psychological characteristics associated with the antisocial or deviant members of our society.

Part II

DIFFERENTIATION OF THE OUT-OF-BODY STATES

Three — DEPERSONALIZATION

This chapter is the first in a series of four in which we will attempt to define further the precise nature of the out-of-body experience while also examining other forms of altered mind/body perception. Our approach in this section is to delineate what an OBE is by demonstrating what it is not. First, we will differentiate it from three pathological conditions—depersonalization, autoscopy, and schizophrenic body boundary disturbances—with which it is commonly confused. Then we will illustrate how it differs from normal altered states of consciousness such as REM dreams, lucid dreams, daydreams, and hypnagogic-hypnopompic states.

Considerable confusion exists in the psychiatric literature concerned with states of consciousness in which there is an altered perception of the mind/body relationship. Related but different terms, such as out-of-body experience, depersonalization, and autoscopic hallucinations, are used interchangeably with a lack of definitional rigor. The problem of variable definition of the syndrome is compounded by the fact that some studies deal with psychiatric or medical patients, others focus on nonpatients, and still others deal with both groups. The fact that some groups of persons with experiences of altered mind/body perception do not define themselves as patients and do not seek treatment, while others do see themselves as in need of help underscores the need for clarification. As we indicated in Chapter Two, Kennedy (1976) refers to out-of-body experiences during meditative practice as "self-induced depersonalization syndrome," even though the experiences lack the essential phenomenological criteria of depersonalization. Sabom (1982) refers to the out-of-body experience during NDE as autoscopic, when clearly the out-of-body experience is different than autoscopic phenomena. These are but two examples of the trend in the literature to confuse these terms. The result is that communication about these experiences and attempts to understand them are confounded. Our intent in our previous work (Gabbard, Twemlow, and Jones 1982) and in our expanded current effort is to bring order and structure to this group of loosely connected human experiences. We are aware that such distinctions must be tentative given the limits of our current state of knowledge, but we feel the attempt is worthwhile because of the differences in treatment implications. There is certainly some overlap among the various syndromes, however, and the distinctions drawn in the ensuing chapters should not be taken as ironclad. We shall begin with the phenomenon of depersonalization.

DEFINITION

The third edition of DSM-III, the American Psychiatric Association's Diagnostic Manual (1980), categorizes depersonalization disorder as a dissociative phenomenon and defines it as an alteration in the perception of the self so that the feeling of one's own reality is temporarily lost. This feeling of unreality may refer to an estrangement from the self, from the body, or from one's surroundings. Derealization refers specifically to the estrangement from one's environment, although derealization is ordinarily part of the depersonalization disorder. Depersonalization may take many forms: one may feel that one's body is dead or numb; one may feel that a certain body part or parts, such as the hands or feet, are not connected with the rest of one's body; one may feel detached from one's self image so that one does not know who one is; or one may have the sense that one is observing oneself at some distance. The latter variant of depersonalization is most commonly confused with out-of-body experience. However, from the foregoing description, it should be clear that the person experiencing depersonalization does not necessarily feel "out-of-body." Noyes et al. (1977) found that the subjective experience of frank detachment from the body is actually infrequent in depersonalization, characterizing only 19 percent of psychiatric patients who suffer from depersonalization.

One of the hallmarks of depersonalization is the subjective

experience of a split between an observing self and a functioning self, even if one does not feel truly separated from one's body. The observing self, from a detached and dispassionate point of view, seems to watch the functioning self behave in an automatic manner. A victim of an automobile accident, for example, may report that he or she experienced the entire accident as though it were happening to someone else, as he or she saw his or her functioning self go through the motions of turning the wheel and stomping on the brakes. A concert pianist in the throes of stage fright may have the feeling he is watching his or her hands dance up and down the keyboard as though they were not his or her own nor under his or her control (Gabbard 1979).

The unreality of depersonalization is further characterized by a barrier between one's self and what one is observing. A dreamlike quality is also present, although the patient is aware that he or she is fully awake and not dreaming. These temporary alterations in reality are common and related to experiences such as deja vu and jamais vu. Nemiah (1980) states that as an isolated and transient experience, depersonalization is not necessarily abnormal and may occur in as many as 50 percent of a given population. He further points out that depersonalization is uncommon as a pure disorder, being found more frequently as a symptom connected with schizophrenia, depression, or anxiety. Fisher and Seidner (1963) studied body experiences in 30 schizophrenic patients, 28 neurotic patients, and 25 normal individuals. There were no significant differences in the incidence of depersonalization between neurotics and schizophrenics. The authors conclude that it is erroneus to assume automatically that a severe psychiatric disturbance is present on the basis of a history of depersonalization. Tucker, Harrow, and Quinlan (1973) confirmed this impression in their report that measures of depersonalization and derealization are similar in several diagnostic categories.

Demographic features of depersonalization, according to Nemiah, include an incidence in women that is twice as great as the incidence in men, and a preference for young people in the age range of 15 to 30, as it is almost unheard of in persons over 40. In over 50 percent of cases, it tends to be a long-lasting chronic condition, while it is merely episodic in the remaining group. All aspects of depersonalization are extremely unpleasant and cause patients to fear that they are going crazy. It is usual for a person who has experienced a depersonalization episode to seek medical attention because of this anxiety. Patients with borderline personality disorders often mutilate themselves as a result of depersonalization experiences, and the fact that they resort to such extreme and self-destructive behavior reflects the intensity of the discomfort produced by depersonalization. The borderline patient who depersonalizes reports that cutting or burning his or her skin reestablishes the sense that his or her body is real, that it is connected with his or her mental self-representation, and that it is responsive to stimuli such as pain.

PSYCHOLOGICAL THEORIES

The perplexing and mysterious phenomenon of depersonalization has attracted the attention of some of history's most brilliant psychoanalytic thinkers for several decades now. Although the explanatory formulations vary considerably, the vast majority of writers view depersonalization as a defense. Freud (1918) described the "Wolf Man's" symptom of depersonalization as a defense against anxiety produced by his wish to return to the womb. Freud himself depersonalized during his famous visit to the Acropolis and later (1936) explained this experience as a defense against the intense oedipally based guilt he felt associated with his success. Fenichel (1945) viewed depersonalization as a defensive measure triggered by an increased narcissistic cathexis of the body or of the mental processes. In other words, depersonalization can be seen as a countercathexis against intense feelings, be they erotic or aggressive, secondary to an intensification of narcissism.

Schilder (1935) stated that, "Depersonalization is a characteristic picture which occurs when an individual does not dare to place his libido either in the outside world or in his own body. The change in the body image results from the withdrawing of libido from the body image" (p. 140). He believed that depersonalization occurs prominently in organs or in environmental objects that have great erotic significance. Vision loses the character of reality, for example, because of the need to deny voyeuristic tendencies. Moreover, the self-observation characteristic of depersonalization is also seen by him as derived from voyeuristic tendencies. The individual punishes himself or herself by not fully seeing the object of desire but substitutes the symbolic equivalent of looking at himself or herself. Nunberg (1932) reported that depersonalization is always a response to loss, particularly a sudden loss of love or the object of love. He saw the feelings of estrangement as the result of a sudden transfer of the libido from the love object to the ego. Bergler and Eidelberg (1935), like Schilder, noted the voyeuristic aspects of self-observation, but they view depersonalization as a defense against anal exhibitionism, which is secondarily transformed into voyeurism in the acceptable form of self-observation.

Rosenfeld (1947) also views depersonalization as a defense, but he sees it as defending against primitive destructive impulses and persecutory anxieties stemming from the paranoid position of infantile development. Blank (1954) shares the view that these anxieties originate from early pregenital fixations, and he explains depersonalization as a defense against anxiety stemming from oral deprivation and oral rage. Stamm (1962) also believes that depersonalization is especially pronounced in persons with deep oral fixations and represents a regressive defensive device. He says it is a return to a primitive, oral, undifferentiated state in which one of the overpowering motives is to withdraw cathexis from external stimuli to relax and to fall asleep.

Jacobson (1959) became interested in depersonalization after studying female prisoners, who depersonalized in response to the trauma of being arrested and taken prisoner by the Nazis in World War II. She says that depersonalization always represents an attempt to solve a narcissistic conflict. However, the narcissistic conflict does not arise from a split between the superego and the ego, but rather from within the ego itself. She views depersonalization as a struggle between conflicting identifications. She describes one patient, for example, whose two contradictory self-images reflected opposing fantasies of identification with a phallic and with a degraded, castrated daughter. She says that unacceptable identifications are defended against by disowning and denying the undesirable part of the ego. In another example of a man who depersonalized during sexual intercourse, she explains the self-observation of this man as a way of absorbing and transforming a sadistic voyeuristic impulse toward the woman by turning it to the self and employing it for denial of identification with a castrated object, that is, the woman with whom he was having intercourse. Sarlin (1962) also conceptualizes depersonalization as defending against conflicting ego identifications. He notes that it may result when a conflict between the individual's parents becomes internalized as two conflicting aspects of the child's ego. The struggle between simultaneous hostile identifications with both parents may cause the individual to lose his or her identity. He said that derealization differs from depersonalization in that cathexis is withdrawn from the object representations and results in feelings of estrangement from others.

Myers (1976) reports that the predominent anxieties he has observed in patients who depersonalize are castration anxiety and the fear of the loss of the object. He says that primarily aggressive drive derivative wishes have to be warded off since they threaten to arouse the two anxieties mentioned previously. He says the observed self-representation may be equated with the phallus. The distancing from the participatory self and the heightened observation of the self serve to ward off the recognition of the participatory self-representation as bad, degraded, or castrated. The duplication of self-representation additionally serves to defend against castration anxiety. He further suggests that primal scene exposure, in which conflicting wishes are aroused to be both intimately involved in, yet distanced from, the exciting and terrifying scene, enhances the predisposition to the later splitting of the self-representation seen in depersonalization. Arlow (1966) holds a similar view that depersonalization involves attributing warded off impulses and the dangerous situation to the participating self, which is then experienced as estranged. In so doing, the individual has evoked an unconscious defensive fantasy in which the dangerous instinctual conflict is viewed as taking place within a stranger rather than within the self. Arlow feels that the patient is not anxious because of the depersonalization, but rather because of the anxiety-arousing danger that produced the depersonalization.

Stolorow (1979) has a somewhat different view of depersonalization phenomena. He points out that the assumption that the splitting of the self is defensive in nature presupposes a prior integration of the self, which may not be accurate when this phenomenon occurs in patients who have experienced early developmental arrest. He holds the opinion that the primitive states of regression characteristic of depersonalization point to arrests in the development of separation-individuation and self-object differentiation. He cites Federn (1952) as the first psychoanalytic thinker to relate these states of estrangement to developmental impairments in self-object boundaries and defects in the sense of self-coherence. He describes a case where a woman depersonalized at each step toward independence through performance of a new activity because these steps confronted her with an experience of separation and differentiation from her mother and, thus, a threatened loss of the symbiotic closeness with the mother. Gabbard (1979) similarly links the depersonalization reaction so common in the performer's stage fright experience with the rapprochement crisis of separation-individuation, that is, the act of performing implies separation-individuation from mother and threatens the performer with withdrawal of mother's love, leading to depersonalization. Elsewhere Gabbard (1983) further elaborates on depersonalization in the stage fright reaction by drawing a link to Kohut's (1977) notion of disintegration anxiety. When the performer feels that the mirroring response from the audience is not forthcoming, this trauma recapitulates an earlier experience of mother's failure to empathically mirror his or her exhibitionistic displays and leads to dissolution of the self, which is experienced physiologically as hyperawareness of some body parts, hypoawareness of others, and an overall sense of lacking cohesion of the body with no control over its functioning.

Both Stolorow (1979) and Gabbard (1979, 1983), then, would argue that depersonalization may be defensive in patients who have attained object constancy and negotiated the oedipal period in a reasonably competent manner, but there may also be instances in which depersonalization is symptomatic of disturbances in the consolidation of a cohesive and stable sense of self. These latter instances are more likely to occur in patients with primitive developmental arrest. Stolorow (1979) asserts that Arlow's comment explaining the anxiety in the depersonalized patient as stemming from instinctual anxiety producing the depersonalization, not from the depersonalization itself, applies only to the higher level patient where depersonalization is truly defensive. He contends that in the developmentally arrested patient, the anxiety is inherent to the depersonalization state itself as it reflects the individual's panic over the fragmenting of his self-representation.

Noyes and Kletti (1976), in their study of accident victims, pointed to the adaptive, lifesaving value of the depersonalization defense. By detaching oneself from the situation and denying that one's body is about to be seriously injured or destroyed, one has a more objective frame of reference from which to find a way out of the situation. For example the mountain climber who falls may have the presence of mind to grab for a ledge and thus save his or her life. In a Darwinian sense, depersonalization may have survival value and therefore can be seen as a positive, adaptive trait.

From the foregoing review of the literature, it should be obvious that depersonalization may have many determinants, in keeping with the core psychoanalytic principle of overdetermination (Waelder 1930), that is, anxieties stemming from several developmental levels converge to form a particular symptom or defense. Genital level anxieties such as castration anxiety are operating at one level, while primitive oral anxieties and even annihilation anxiety operate at more primitive levels. Moreover, depersonalization may originate in certain persons as an experience of dissolution of the self without any defensive function whatsoever. One or more of these determinants may be active in a particular individual's depersonalization experience, and the particular determinant will obviously vary from individual to individual, depending on the psychological constellation of the particular person. We will consider this concept of causation in detail in Chapter Eleven. Three clinical examples will illustrate the varying origins of the phenomenon.

CASE 1

Miss D. was a 19-year-old woman who came to treatment because of serious and uncontrollable self-mutilating tendencies and chronic suicidal thoughts. As her history unfolded, it became clear that she had been involved in incestuous sexual relations with her step-father since the age of eight and had only recently stopped such behavior. She had started experiencing depersonalization at the age of eight, when the sexual involvement began, and had gone in and out of episodes of estrangement ever since that time. The depersonalization clearly served a defensive function to her. When her step-father would begin physical contact with her, the anxiety created by that sexual contact was so great that she would find herself observing the sexual interaction as a spectator from across the room. She said she could look at her body if she chose to, but usually did not since the sight of sexual activity with the step-father was so repugnant to her. Her body seemed unreal to her, and she compared it to a "rubber mannequin." She fell into this defensive pattern each time her step-father molested her. Eventually, the depersonalization would occur spontaneously in other situations, such as a family argument at the dinner table or any other situation where stress or anxiety was prominent. By the time she was 19 and came for psychiatric treatment, depersonalization was a chronic state, in which she felt dead and unreal much of the time. When she cut on her forearms, she felt tremendous relief from this unpleasant depersonalized state. The pain of the cut was preferable to the estrangement, and it reassured her that she was real and had a body that was her own.

In Miss D., the defensive function of the depersonalization could be stated as follows: "That is not me who is experiencing the sexual molestation. That is not my body, because I am over here in another part of the room watching it happen to a stranger." The sexual activity could then be attributed to a bad, degraded self which was split off and not part of her. Moreover, through depersonalization, she was able to defend against her own instinctual pleasure inherent in the gratification of the oedipal wish. The body for this patient became the instrument of gratification of forbidden incestuous pleasures, so that the chronic state of depersonalization was an unconscious way in which Miss D. disavowed any connection between her self-representation and her body, with its degraded and unacceptable properties. The depersonalization may, in fact, have been lifesaving since the patient felt increasingly suicidal as she got in touch with this splitting of the self through psychotherapy. The more she integrated these disavowed parts of her, the more she felt that she was unacceptable and deserved to die.

CASE 2

Dr. E. was a 53-year-old Jewish surgeon, who was born in Germany and fled at the age of nine, when Hitler began his campaign to exterminate the Jews. He lived in the United States for many years and did not return to his hometown in Germany until he was 53. When he visited the house in which he had grown up and the cemetery in which his relatives were buried, he depersonalized. Dr. E. experienced the events as though they were not happening to him. He said it was dreamlike and that it felt as though an invisible barrier existed between him and the objects in his environment. He had the sense that he was not really there and that, in his words, "I was me, but I was not me at the same time."

As Dr. E. reflected on these experiences, it became clear that conflicting ego identifications were operating. His experience of himself as the persecuted young Jewish boy and as the successful surgeon in the United States were difficult to integrate. Moreover, the powerful affects associated with his memories of that town threatened to overwhelm him. The pain and the outrage he felt at the knowledge that three-quarters of his family had been murdered in the holocaust threatened to flood his ego, so that the depersonalization defense also served the purpose of warding off those intense affects.

He could view the experience as not really happening to him, and thereby disavow that his roots were really in that particular place. Hence, those tragic memories did not occur, and he did not need to react to them. Finally, he could also disavow the survivor guilt accompanying the realization that he had made it out of Germany while others in his family had not.

CASE 3

Mrs. F. was a 33-year-old housewife who came to treatment on the verge of a psychotic decompensation that was being defended against through the use of obsessive-compulsive defenses. Her presenting complaint was that she was consumed with guilt about her five-year-old son's illness. When he had been 16-months old, he had contracted encephalitis and had subsequently developed a seizure disorder. Her entire life revolved around catering to this boy and trying to relieve herself of the feeling that she had been responsible for the encephalitis, although there was no evidence that she had any real responsibility for his contracting the illness. She went through a number of mental and behavioral rituals as a way of warding off her anxiety and impending psychotic decompensation. She started group psychotherapy, which in retrospect may not have been the appropriate treatment modality for her. She entered a group that had been in process for approximately three-and-a-half years with a fairly stable membership. The patients were advanced in their working through of their various neurotic issues, and at the point where she entered the group, the themes were focusing on oedipal issues and particularly on incestuous sexual fantasies. Mrs. F. found this material quite disturbing. She became alarmed that either her father had had sexual feelings toward her or she had had sexual feelings toward him at the time she reached puberty.

She seemed to have a rather thin repression barrier, as this material surfaced too rapidly without appropriate defenses being brought to bear. The therapist became concerned that she had too ready access to this material, but it was too late. She began to decompensate into a psychotic state. Between group therapy sessions, she called the therapist and asked to see him in a private consultation. She reported misperceiving things at her house. She felt that she was dead and had left her body. This state of depersonalization was particularly interesting since she wondered if she was having an out-of-body experience. However, she could not actually see her body from a point distant in space. Rather, she simply felt like her body must have died, and her mind was alive but was not connected to her body. She repeatedly expressed concern about the possibility that she had committed sexual acts with her father and with her son, both of which were unfounded in reality. She also was anxious about the possibility that she had touched her son in a sexual way while changing his diaper.

With the help of antipsychotic medication and antidepressant medication, she reorganized, and her psychotic symptoms went into remission. However, she continued to have occasional episodes of depersonalization, although of less severity than those occurring during her psychotic state. She was terminated from the group therapy and changed to individual therapy of a supportive variety since this process would prevent her from being assaulted by sexual issues that she was not capable of processing or defending against. She ultimately had a reasonably good outcome despite periodic bouts of depersonalization.

This example of depersonalization illustrates how the phenomenon can accompany the prodrome or the onset of a psychotic episode. As with Miss D., the depersonalization served the function of detaching herself from a body that was viewed as an instrument of incestuous sexuality. However, while Miss D. had sufficient ego strength to maintain reality testing and see the defensive aspects of this process, Mrs. F.'s ego was overwhelmed by the incestuous material and it fragmented into a psychotic state. Her comment that her body was dead was a psychotic denial that her body, with all its unacceptable impulses of a sexual nature, even existed. Relevant historical information included the report that at age 12 she became obsessed with the idea that everything her father touched would become contaminated with her germs. This led to a compulsion to wash doorknobs or anything else her father may have touched. At this same age the patient began menstruating. Projective psychological testing indicated profound ego weaknesses typical of lower-level borderline ego organization with predominantly obsessive-compulsive defenses to ward off decompensation. The testing also indicated that the patient was in a developmental crisis in which the evaluation of her current situation was quite discrepant with earlier ambitions. Instead of being out in the world as she originally had hoped, she found herself very much hemmed in and trapped, taking care of a sick child. Numerous phallic images on the Rorschach included arrow-

Table 3.1
COMPARISON OF DEPERSONALIZATION AND OBE

Depersonalization	OBE
Observing self watches functioning self	Observing self and functioning self are experienced as one (physical body is inactive)
Usually does not feel "out-of-body"	Must feel "out-of-body" by definition
Experienced as dreamlike	Not experienced as dreamlike
Typically unpleasant	Typically pleasant
Affects: anxiety, panic, emptiness	Affects: joy, ecstasy, feelings of calm, peace and quiet
Often stress-induced (sympathetic)	Usually relaxation-induced (parasympathetic)
Experienced as pathological and strange	Experienced as religious, spiritual and noetic
Age distribution 15–30; rarely over 40	No characteristic age group
Sex distribution 2:1 female	Even sex distribution

heads, totem poles, guns, rockets, and sharp daggers. These images reflected a partial unconscious identification with men and masculine things in rejection of more feminine interests. Hence, there was also evidence that conflicting ego identifications may have contributed to the pathogenesis of depersonalization in this patient.

DEPERSONALIZATION VERSUS OBE

Now that we have defined and illustrated the depersonalization phenomenon, we can outline the main differences between depersonalization and out-of-body experience to help the clinician differentiate the two states of altered mind/body perception. Table 3.1 summarizes these differences. First of all, the characteristic split between an observing and a functioning self, which is one of the hallmarks of depersonalization, is not found in OBE, where the observing self and the functioning self are experienced more like one combined entity located with the subject's consciousness outside his physical body. The physical body is itself inactive and nonfunctional —that is, in a relaxed state, such as sitting in a chair or lying on a bed.

A second differential point, as mentioned previously, is that depersonalizers do not necessarily feel physically outside of their bodies. They may simply feel their bodies as dead, numb, or unreal. Only 19 percent of psychiatric patients with depersonalization and only 26 percent of accident victims who depersonalize experience frank detachment from the body (Noyes et al. 1977). In contrast the OBE seems to be a more specific experience: by definition, the subject must have the feeling that his or her mind has separated from his or her body at a distance. A third differential point is that one of the common feelings in depersonalization is the feeling of unreality often described as "dreamlike." On the other hand almost all subjects report out-of-body experience to be "more real than a dream." Many persons who have had an out-of-body experience emphasize repeatedly that their experience was as real and as clear as the waking state.

The affective state of the individual accounts for a fourth differential point. Nemiah (1980) notes that the experience of depersonalization is unpleasant in every way and often motivates the patient to seek medical help. Selinsky (1968) also points out that persons undergoing depersonalization describe their state of feeling as one of discomfort, uneasiness, and even great anxiety. Both Nemiah and Selinsky call attention to the frequent feeling of impending disintegration or the belief that one is "going crazy." Out-of-body experience, on the other hand, is more typically characterized by feelings of calm, peace and quiet, joy, and ecstasy. As indicated in Chapter One, fear is relatively uncommon among persons having OBE, and the belief that one is "going crazy" is rare.

Some controversy exists in the literature on depersonalization concerning the precipitating factors. Selinsky notes that they are often reactions that accompany acute and intense anxiety. Ackner (1954) maintains that depersonalization can be triggered by sensory isolation, fatigue, drugs, and certain physiologic changes. Roberts (1960), in a study of normal students, noted that fatigue, in association with other conditions such as nervousness, danger, menstruation, and high temperature is commonly present. Noyes and Kletti (1976), Noyes et al. (1977), and Gabbard (1979, 1983) have all linked depersonalization to situations of anxiety and hyperarousal. Noyes et al. conclude that anxiety is clearly of etiological significance: the syndrome appears very similar in normal persons exposed to danger and in psychiatric patients during the symptomatic period of their illness, suggesting a degree of uniformity irrespective of the substrate from which it arises.

A review of the literature, then, suggests at least a trend designating depersonalization as associated with a hyperaroused anxiety state, where sympathetic activation is more predominant than parasympathetic in the autonomic nervous system. In contrast OBE subjects infrequently report emotional stress as a precipitating factor, and nearly 80 percent describe the pre-OBE state as one of mental calmness and physical relaxation, suggesting a predominantly parasympathetic activation.

Another differential point is the fact that depersonalization is experienced as pathological and strange. Out-of-body experience, on the other hand, is often perceived as a religious, spiritual, and noetic phenomenon akin to mystical or religious conversion experiences. This mystical quality is one of the central differentiating factors between depersonalization and OBE and may account for the fact that persons having OBE do not ordinarily see themselves as in need of psychiatric attention. In our sample we performed univariate independent group t-tests on our data. This analysis indicated that subjects who experience fear were significantly less likely to experience that episode as spiritual or religious in nature (dF=302, p .0138) than those who experience no fear. Those who experience fear may have been reporting depersonalization rather than out-of-body experience. On the other hand, because of beliefs about the relationship of mind and body, persons with an OBE may have some secondary concerns about the experience that lead them to seek reassurance that they are not emotionally disturbed or psychotic.

Finally, there are demographic differences between the two states. The age distribution of OBE appears to be quite different from that of depersonalization. Nemiah (1980) notes that depersonalization is a disorder of younger people, starting commonly between the ages of 15 and 30 and almost never present in patients over 40. The OBE, on the other hand, is evenly distributed from the ages of two to 65 without any clustering whatsoever around particular age groups. Also, depersonalization is twice as common in females, while OBE shows no sex preference, according to our data.

While depersonalization may seem more clearly defensive than OBE, both may actually serve defensive functions. The similarities and differences of this aspect of the experiences will be discussed in Chapter Eleven.

TREATMENT

Systematic clinical studies on the treatment of depersonalization do not exist. Occasional episodes of depersonalization require little more than reassurance as to the nature of the symptom. For the more chronic varieties of depersonalization disorder, it is unclear whether psychotherapy is useful or not (Nemiah 1980). Ambrosino (1973) makes the clinical observation that imipramine and desipramine are often very effective in the management of depersonalization states while phenothiazines and possibly electroconvulsive therapy may actually aggravate the condition. When depersonalization accompanies a major psychotic episode, a combination of tricyclic antidepressants and antipsychotic medication may be helpful, as in the case of Mrs. F. above. In most cases treatment is determined according to the context in which the depersonalization occurs, that is, coexisting illnesses, ego strengths, presence or absence of psychosis, motivation for psychotherapy, and similar patient attibutes that may not be directly related to the depersonalization symptom. Occasionally, depersonalization constitutes part of the aura preceding a seizure, particularly in the temporal lobe area. In these cases, of course, appropriate antiseizure medication, such as diphenylhydantoin (Dilantin), may be useful.

Four — AUTOSCOPY: THE DOPPELGÄNGER AND BEYOND

In the late nineteenth century, Heinrich Heine wrote a poem that was beautifully set to music by Franz Schubert in the Schwanengesang. It was called, "Der Doppelgänger":

The night is quiet, the streets are still;
Here in this house my dear one used to live.
She has left the town long since,
But the house still stands in the same square.

Another man stands there too, and stares into the sky,
And wrings his hands with the weight of his grief.
I am filled with horror when I see his face —
The moon shows me my own features.

You ghostly double! You pale companion!
Why do you ape the pain of love
That tortured me in this place,
Full many a night in time gone by?

Heine's poem is only one example of the nineteenth century literary fascination with the phenomenon of the doppelgänger, that is, the double. The notion of seeing one's double is not only a literary metaphor, but also a clinical syndrome. Autoscopy, also known as heautoscopy, autoscopic hallucinations, and autoscopic phenomena, literally means "seeing one's self," if we examine the word from the standpoint of its etymological origins. While the theme of the double is pervasive in nineteenth century Romantic literature, clinical reports of autoscopic phenomena in the scientific literature are much rarer. Earlier this century, papers surfaced from European sources (Sollier 1903; Bogaert 1934; Menninger-Lerchenthal 1935; Lhermitte 1951), while the definitive paper on the subject comes from Lukianowicz (1958) of the United Kingdom. In this paper he describes seven cases of autoscopic phenomena, in which the patient sees an image or apparition of himself or herself appearing suddenly in front of him or her, as though it were reflected in a mirror. Lukianowicz goes on to say that these phantoms are occasionally perceived in other sensory spheres besides the visual—the subject may "hear" his or her image "speak," he or she may perceive the phantom's movements as though they were his own, and he may even experience the double as an emotional part of himself or herself. Hence Lukianowicz comes up with the following definition: "Autoscopy is a complex psychosensorial hallucinatory perception of one's own body image projected into the external visual space" (1958, p. 199).

Defined narrowly and specifically as in Lukianowicz' paper, autoscopy is a rare clinical syndrome. However, the literature on autoscopic hallucinations is inextricably linked with the more general phenomenon of the double as it exists in psychopathological experiences, in literature, in art, and in everyday life. In this chapter we will first focus on the double in literature and in anthropology to serve as a background for understanding the psychological meaning and significance of autoscopic phenomena. Then we will discuss the specific clinical syndrome described by Lukianowicz and explore the etiology of the syndrome from both an organic and a psychodynamic standpoint. Finally, we will differentiate the experience of autoscopy from the out-of-body experience.

HISTORICAL ORIGINS OF THE DOUBLE

As with so many other literary themes, the first references to the double can be found in classical Greek literature. The origin of the double is poetically described by Aristophanes in Plato's *Symposium*. Before the appearance of human beings as we know them, so the story goes, a noble race of creatures existed who had four arms, four legs, and two heads. They moved themselves by cartwheels rather than by walking in an upright position. Their temerity led them to launch an effort to climb Mt. Olympus, endeavoring to reach the gods. The gods were infuriated at their hubris and retaliated by cleaving them into two separate beings. These miserable creatures, so the legend continues, are engaged in a never-ending search for their soulmates, that is, their other halves. An additional reference to Greek literature comes from Lhermitte (1951), who cites a story by Aristotle of a man who could not go for a walk without seeing his own image coming toward him.

The classical psychoanalytic monograph on the double was written by Otto Rank (1914), in which he exhaustively surveys both the anthropological-cultural and the mythological-literary themes of the double. In examining various folk beliefs about the double, Rank notes the connection between the fantasies about one's shadow and the notion of the double. He cites the German provincial belief that stepping on one's own shadow is a sign of death. He says that the superstitions about one's shadow are closely related to beliefs about guardian spirits. Folk mythology is replete with ideas about one's guardian angel joining one's shadow and beliefs that the double who catches sight of himself or herself must die within a year. The inhabitants of Anboyna and Uliase, two islands on the equator, do not leave their houses at noon because in this location, their shadows disappear, and the belief prevalent among these islanders is that they will lose their souls along with the disappearance of their shadows. Hence, there is some equivalence between the human soul and the shadow in many cultural mythologies. The Fiji islanders, for example, believe that every person has two souls—a bright one that exists in one's reflection on the surface of water or in a mirror and that remains nearby the place of death, and a dark one that exists in one's shadow and is consigned to eternal damnation following death. Rank points out that the devil, according to Russian beliefs, has no shadow because he is an evil spirit. Similarly, those who make contracts with the devil are reported not to have shadows. Linked to this idea is the folk belief that vampires cast no shadow and have no mirror images. As these personifications of evil have no soul and no reflection, they are deprived of the possibility of eternal salvation. The connection between the double and the soul is clear in these beliefs and may account for the association of the double with death.

Rank elegantly documents this pervasive link between death and the double, a cross-cultural connection that is striking. The superstition, for instance, that one will die if one allows one's portrait to be painted can be found in peoples of Germany, Greece, Russia, Albania, England, and Scotland. Even in ancient Greece, there was reportedly a rule not to gaze into one's reflection on the water as that would result in death. A similar belief regarding having one's photograph taken is present among Eskimos, central African tribes, American Indians, East Indians, and various Asian people. The fantasy here is that if someone possesses an image on a picture, the soul of the person being photographed is possessed by that photographic image, and this transfer of the soul can have a harmful or deadly effect upon the subject. Rank also examines the myth of Narcissus in light of this theme and points out that Tiresias was asked at the birth of Narcissus if the child could expect a long life. The prophet replied that his longevity was dependent on his not seeing himself. Narcissus, of course, did in fact take his own life after becoming entranced by his reflection.

The nineteenth and early twentieth century, as mentioned previously, are replete with references to doubles. Rank (1914), Coleman (1934), Lhermitte (1951), Dewhurst (1954), and Grotstein (1982, 1983) have all reviewed and interpreted this literature at some length. We will touch on a few examples here.

In Joseph Conrad's *The Secret Sharer* a clandestine stowaway on a ship serves as a kind of alter ego of one of the sailors. This double seems to be the container of various qualities that are split off and unacceptable to the protagonist of the story. Conrad's fascination with the double apparently stems from his own doppelgänger experiences with Bertrand Russell and with Ford Madox Hueffer (Hamilton 1979). Russell and Conrad had an immediate and intense attraction to one another upon their first meeting. Russell describes it as follows: "We looked into each other's eyes, half-appalled and half-intoxicated to find ourselves together in such a region. The emotion was as intense as passionate love and at the same time all embracing.... in something very fundamental, we were extraordinarily at one" (1956, p. 89). This unusual response to one another is an example of the doppelgänger phenomenon, according to Hamilton (1979), who links it to the commonality of early loss of both parents, an historical factor in the lives of both men. Hamilton points out that Freud and the Viennese playwright Arthur Schnitzler had a similar kind of relationship. Both of these men had very similar early childhood experiences as well. Hamilton believes that the specific doubling described in *The Secret Sharer* was based on an actual friendship between Conrad and his friend and fellow writer of 11 years, Ford Madox Hueffer. Hence, Conrad's doppelgänger experiences in real life, as well as a number of depersonalization episodes (Hamilton 1975), may have contributed to his literary fascination with the theme of the double.

Hamilton's use of the term doppelgänger in the context of the special relationship between Conrad and Russell illustrates one of the problems with the highly personalized usage of the concept. Clearly, Hamilton recognizes that neither Russell nor Conrad literally thought he was seeing his own double. He is using the term doppelgänger to describe a profound sense of oneness or sameness felt by both men, a kind of "love at first sight" stemming from the perception, accurate or otherwise, that each possessed similar qualities. The immediacy and intensity of the experience is reminiscent of a transference reaction in psychotherapy or psychoanalysis, where each is attributing to the other a variety of qualities that may or may not be present. Indeed, Kohut (1971) writes of the therapeutic activation of these kinds of narcissistic transferences in psychoanalysis. More specifically, he refers to a particular form of transference called the alter ego transference or twinship. In his own words, "The narcissistically cathected object is experienced as being like the grandiose self or being very similar to it...dreams, and especially fantasies, referring to a relationship with such an alter ego or twin (or conscious wishes for such a relationship) are frequently encountered in the analysis of narcissistic personalities" (1971, p. 115). Hence, the special kinship between Conrad and Russell may best be explained as a narcissistic transference reaction where the primitive grandiose self of each was hungering for mirroring and found it in this special relationship. The broad usage of doppelgänger as descriptive of this phenomenon underscores the need to clarify how the term is being used in any given context.

Other variations of the double theme include Oscar Wilde's novel, *The Picture of Dorian Gray*, in which the handsome young Gray is granted the narcissistic wish never to age; all signs of growing old are transferred to the portrait on the wall. As this portrait ages, Gray is filled with revulsion at his mirror image and ends his life by stabbing the picture, resulting in an instantaneous reversal of himself and the portrait as he falls dead with the knife in his heart. Edgar Allan Poe used the theme in his story, *William Wilson*, where the main character meets his double as a child. This double shares the same name and resembles Wilson in every other aspect. The only difference is in the fact that the double's voice cannot rise above a whisper.

The counterpart is perceived only by Wilson himself and goes unseen by his companions.

A variant on the subject is provided in the well-known *Doctor Jekyll and Mr. Hyde* by Robert Louis Stevenson. The doubling phenomenon in this story reflects an intrapsychic splitting process, where opposite selves, one good and one bad, occupy the same psyche. This motif is emblematic of the psychological wish to deny and split off unacceptable and impulse-ridden parts of one's self by attributing them to another person. Famous nineteenth-century French writers, such as Baudelaire, Stendahl, Rimbaud, and others, have demonstrated the importance of splitting off the creative part of themselves from the part bound by the social and literary mores of the day. In that era even slight deviations from prescribed literary styles and routines were not tolerated by the literary establishment. It was left to a group of mavericks, including Chauteaubriand and Flaubert, as well as those mentioned previously, to break free from these shackles and produce the seminal psychological themes of modern literature. They were able to accomplish this creative leap by virtue of their capacity to split off a part of themselves that was capable of writing in a free and uninhibited manner.

Many other literary examples of the doppelgänger phenomenon could be cited, including Dostoyevsky's monumental work, *The Double*, *Notturno* by d'Annunzio, Kafka's *The Trial*, and some of the works of Goethe, who, as we note in the Introduction, had an autoscopic experience himself. The double theme is pervasive in the writings of E.T.A. Hoffman, particularly in his short stories, "Story of the Lost Reflection," and "The Doubles." The stories of De Maupassant, especially *La Horla*, are other well-known literary sources. Rank (1914) details the lives of several of these authors, including Hoffman, Poe, Maupassant, Heine, and Dostoyevsky, pointing to the fact that they spent much of their lives afflicted with serious neurological or psychiatric disorders. He asserts that their interest in the doppelgänger theme stems from similarities in psychopathology. He states: "The pathological disposition toward psychological disturbances is conditioned to a large degree by the splitting of the personality, with special emphasis upon the ego-complex, to which corresponds an abnormally strong interest in one's own person, his psychic states, and his destiny" (p. 48). Rank is somewhat unconvincing in his effort to lump together a variety of psychopathological syndromes and to assert their essential similarity, not to mention his use of a highly controversial technique of literary criticism, in which the critic assumes that a distant and "wild" analysis of the biographical data of the author will explain the themes in the author's works.

AUTOSCOPY AS A CLINICAL SYNDROME

The clinical phenomenon of autoscopy has a much narrower definition than the broad usage of the idea of the double in literature and in mythology. Wigan first introduced the term into the medical literature (Lhermitte 1948) when he described a patient who could summon and actually see a double of himself. Sollier (1903) published a classical treatment of the subject at the beginning of this century in France. Lukianowicz (1958) described and defined autoscopic phenomena in some detail, lending some coherence and diagnostic rigor to the clinical picture. He reports seven cases of autoscopic phenomena, which allow him to derive specific criteria that are characteristic for the diagnosis. These cases make fascinating reading, and we will supply one here for the sake of illustration.

Lukianowicz describes a 56-year-old retired schoolteacher who had experienced autoscopic hallucinations ever since her husband's funeral. One day she returned from the cemetery in the twilight of the late afternoon and noticed a lady in front of her in her bedroom. As the teacher looked at her right hand to turn on the light, the phantom lady made the same movement with her left hand as though she were a mirror image. The double was dressed in an identical fashion. Despite the bizarre nature of this situation, the teacher was not shocked nor fearful, but she essentially felt the absence of any feeling. As she undressed, her phantom counterpart undressed in the same manner. She felt that this "second self" was more alive and emotionally warm than she herself was. When she closed her eyes, she lost sight of the phantom. Since that particular evening, this woman had had almost daily visits from her double, particularly around dusk. She would see it only when she looked straight ahead and typically lost sight of it when she turned her head. The image was life-sized, but the most distinct part of it were the face, torso, and hands. The phantom was described as misty and transparent. Somehow, the schoolteacher felt that she "knew" and "felt" the exact position in space of the phantom's legs. Lukianowicz refers to this as kinesthetic perception. He also emphasizes the fact that the patient had insight into the unreality of the double. She realized it was only an hallucination, but nevertheless, she felt it was an integral part of herself.

From this case and the six others, Lukianowicz derives the following characteristics of autoscopic phenomena: 1) the phantom double ordinarily appears suddenly to the subject, without advance warning; 2) certain patients with seizure disorders or migraine headaches may have an autoscopic experience before, instead of, or after an attack; 3) normally, the autoscopic double appears only as the face or a face and torso—it is uncommon for the entire body to be well visualized; 4) the image is usually seen clearly and with all the details of a mirror image; 5) the double is ordinarily colorless and transparent; 6) in most cases the phantom imitates all the movements, and particularly the facial expressions, of the "original"; 7) it is common for the subject to perceive the double with more than just the visual senses—kinesthetic, intellectual, emotional, and auditory perception are possible accompaniments of the visual perception; 8) the most frequent emotional reaction associated with seeing the autoscopic image is sadness, although bewilderment may also be present; 9) a peculiar form of detached insight into the unreality of the experience is present in most cases; 10) the double is most frequently localized in the visual space directly in front of the subject, about a yard away; 11) the experience generally lasts a few seconds at a time and may occur with a frequency of once in a lifetime to a continual presence; 12) dusk is the most common time of appearance of the phantoms; 13) demographic factors such as sex, intelligence, education, and age seem to play no role in subjects who experience autoscopy; and 14) there does not seem to be a causal relationship between autoscopy and psychosis.

Damas Mora et al. (1980) report a case and discuss the classification of the phenomenon in a recent British paper. They advocate the use of the term "heautoscopy" since an autoscope is an instrument that has become connected in medical terminology with laryngology. They emphasize that the important feature of these experiences is the psychological identity between the subject and the vision, rather than the vision itself, and aver that the feeling of belonging associated with the image is critical. They report a case of a young man who repeatedly saw a vision of himself so vividly that he even jumped into a river to save the double when he thought it was drowning. He eventually became suicidal because of the frequent visions of his double. The double talked, and he could recognize his own voice. The phantom appeared when the young man was under stress, and on every occasion he experienced the feeling of impending disaster and often feared becoming controlled by the double. During one hospital admission, there was clear evidence of thought insertion and thought withdrawal. After being diagnosed and treated for paranoid schizophrenia, he improved, but he continued to hallucinate occasionally. The double continued to appear to him over a period of more than 10 years. It had a helpless expression and would appear in his visual field between 3 feet and 20 yards from him. He also noted that the phantom moved away when he tried to approach it or touch it. Following treatment with electroconvulsive therapy and medication, he was able to function well and required no medication for a period of four years at follow up.

Damas Mora et al. review much of the Spanish literature on the subject and argue that autoscopy is not a unitary phenomenon. They point out that Alonso-Fernandez (1976) asserts that it is a syndrome with wide variations. Alonso-Fernandez considers there to be three clinical forms: a form involving depersonalization, a hallucinatory form, and a delusional form.

A recent U.S. contribution to the clinical literature is that of Faguet (1979), who reports three cases and emphasizes the importance of illness, injury, and hospitalization as precipitants of the syndrome. He cites a case of a physician who was admitted to the hospital and awoke to a transparent image of himself at the bedside. A diabetic female patient spoke of ghostly visitations at night during her hospitalization. A third autoscopic case involved a 24-year-old artist who was admitted to the hospital for the first time after sustaining trauma in a car accident. As she was waiting for her x-ray, she saw an image of herself enter the room, and she fainted. Faguet believes that these isolated autoscopic hallucinations are not necessarily pathognomonic of any particular illness, but are more likely unusual reactions to stress or fatigue.

ORGANIC CAUSES

In considering the etiology of autoscopy, the literature can be divided between the organic theories and the psychological theories. A fair number of autoscopic cases occur in association with documented brain pathology. These reports suggest irritative lesions in the temporo-parieto-occipital areas, as Menninger-Lerchenthal (1935) first discerned 50 years ago. However, as Lukianowicz (1958) and Damas Mora et al. (1980) point out, there is considerable disagreement in the literature as to the value of and justification for localizing such complex hallucinatory phenomena to certain brain areas. Lukianowicz (1958) notes that a considerable number of autoscopic patients suffer from seizure disorders and/or migraine headaches. Damas Mora et al. have made an exhaustive search of the literature for organic etiologies of autoscopy, producing the following list of reported associations between organic illness and autoscopy:* seizure disorder, migraine, toxic-confusional states of typhus and influenza, encephalitis, posttraumatic cerebral lesions, labyrinthine disorders, terminal cancer, pulmonary tuberculosis and intestinal hemorrhage, alcoholic and drug intoxication, hypophyseal tumor, subarachnoid hemorrhage, bulbar hemorrhage, and postelectroconvulsive confusion. They also note that reports of autoscopy occurring in apparently normal individuals are often in connection with physiological stress states such as anxiety, fatigue, or exhaustion.

In the first known report of autoscopy in the medical literature, Wigan (1844) related the phenomenon to a splitting of the functions of the two cerebral hemispheres. Dewhurst and Pearson (1955) report three patients with clear brain pathology, including one with a vascular lesion in the brain, one with a left temporal tumor, and one with a cortical injury from shrapnel. They note, however, that a purely neurological explanation is not adequate to explain the complexity and variability of the phenomena. In our own experience we have come across one case of a patient with a temporal lobe seizure disorder, who had vivid out-of-body experiences as part of his aura. In reviewing the literature on autoscopy, one must wonder to what extent some of these reports are actually out-of-body experiences rather than true autoscopic phenomena. More will be said about the differential diagnosis of the two later in the chapter.

PSYCHOLOGICAL CAUSES

Lukianowicz (1958) recognizes the existence of idiopathic autoscopy, that is, those experiences occurring in states without known brain pathology, and he suggests that these reports argue in favor of a psychological theory of etiology. Rank (1914) notes that the occurrence of these phenomena in the primitive as well as in the cultured and educated neurotic could be explained by the fact that

---

*The reader is reminded here that association in time does not necessarily imply a cause-effect relationship.

both share the terror of death and the magical belief in immortality. He says that there is a powerful narcissistic wish to avoid self-extinction that manifests itself in the belief in souls and in eternal life following death of the physical body. The appearance of the double then is a defensive reassurance to the individual that a second life, indeed a second self, exists that will not be threatened by death. Freud devoted considerable attention to the phenomenon of the double in his 1919 paper on "The Uncanny." Anticipating the development of the structural theory in psychoanalysis only a few years later, Freud connected experiences of seeing one's double to an intrapsychic agency, the conscience, which serves the function of self-observation and self-criticism. He argued for a division between this critical agency and the rest of the ego. Upon seeing his own reflection, Freud experienced a sense of the uncanny along with a profound dislike for his image. Certain split-off and unacceptable parts of one's self are projected onto this image and disavowed as something foreign, resulting in a distaste for the image, according to Freud. Freud also shared Rank's view that the double experience harkens back to a stage of primary narcissism and serves as a defense against death and dissolution of the self.

Ostow (1960) notes the fact that these experiences have been reported autobiographically by a number of normal, even distinguished, individuals, such as Archbishop Frederick and the physicist Ernst Mach. He connects autoscopy with rebirth as well as with death. He says that in his clinical cases, a depressive withdrawal of object and self-cathexis occurs followed by a retreat into primary narcissism. In a state of ego depletion, ego splitting occurs, resulting in autoscopic experience. He asserts that the combination of the collapse into primary narcissism and the state of ego depletion, however, are not sufficient conditions in themselves for the occurrence of autoscopic phenomena. In addition to these elements, he insists that there must be a tendency preexisting in the patient for the ego to split into acting and observing fragments. He is quick to point out, however, that autoscopy is paradoxically not really an instance of self-observation. Rather, it is a magical process by which an image of the self is rejected instead of the real self, in the same way as primitive man kills an adversary by employing an effigy. He shares Freud's idea (1919) that the image of the self is disliked, as it is a projected and repudiated portion of one's self.

Faguet (1979) notes the common restitutive function of the hallucinations in his three cases. He feels they recapture an important object relation, that is, the image of one's self as it had been or still could possibly be. His hospitalized patients were under extraordinary stress as well as suffering the narcissistic injury of being hospitalized and dependent. This regressed state may result in the wish-fulfilling vision of one's self as one was before and would again like to be.

Of all the psychoanalytic writing on the subject of autoscopy, none is more thought-provoking and comprehensive in its treatment of the subject than the writings of Grotstein (1982, 1983). He feels autoscopic phenomena are much more pervasive than would be indicated by the narrow definition of Lukianowicz. In his own words: "If we were to expand the definition of autoscopy to include such ultrasensual phenomena as fantasies (intrapsychic experiences), we might say then that autoscopic phenomena include the whole spectrum of self-consciousness, 'normal' through 'abnormal.' The 'sensual band' (visual, kinesthetic, and auditory) of autoscopy proper would then be located on one position of the spectrum. We could then state that autoscopy seems to be a manifestation of a difficulty in the *tone* of narcissistic well-being and reveals a state of *alienation*" (1982, p. 73). In his two papers he reports some 13 clinical vignettes illustrating a variety of psychological phenomena, including dreams, vivid visual fantasies, true autoscopic hallucinations (in the narrow sense), depersonalization episodes, out-of-body experiences, and even a near-death experience. Recognizing that all of these experiences are not phenomenologically similar, Grotstein, nonetheless, seeks to illustrate that they have common underlying mechanisms. Under this broadened definition, he maintains that these basic etiological mechanisms may occur in normals, where the experience of doubling has no pathological significance, and is equally apt to occur in psychotics, borderline patients, and those with organic brain disturbances.

Grotstein acknowledges the complexity of autoscopic phenomena and makes it clear that only a model based on the principle of multidetermination does full justice to the richness and variability of the syndrome. He understands autoscopy as involving four essential mechanisms.

1. Splitting of consciousness and a projective identification (that is, externalization) of one's body image is, in his view, central to the autoscopic phenomena. Grotstein asserts that autoscopy is the "sensory epitome of self-consciousness," and from that standpoint the experience reveals certain emotional attitudes of the subject

toward the double or observed self. He notes that these attitudes are generally critical ones and explains this as stemming from the fact that the double is a projective identification, that is, a disavowal of unacceptable parts of one's self. This helps us understand the aforementioned negative reaction of Freud to seeing his reflection as well as Wilde's *Dorian Gray* and Stevenson's *Jekyll and Hyde* stories, in which bad and unwanted parts of the self are split-off and projectively disavowed by attributing them to a double. Grotstein discusses this in terms of the uncanny feeling connected with autoscopy. This feeling stems from the fear of the return of the repressed, as the phantom in autoscopy represents an example of the return of a disavowed and split-off, if not repressed, self.

2. The split-brain phenomenon is viewed by Grotstein as another determinant of autoscopic experiences. He notes that the corpus callosum and the deep cerebral commisures connecting the two hemispheres of the brain do not myelinate until around four to five months of age. Myelination is not completed until adolescence. From a developmental perspective, then, Grotstein argues that the infant experiences two separate minds, a left hemispheric organization and a right hemispheric organization, which only gradually come together with maturity. Hence autoscopy, in Grotstein's view, may be secondary to a breakdown of the interhemispheric coordination and integration, what he calls "interhemispheric diplopia." Altered states of consciousness, such as fugue states, dreams, seizures, drug intoxication, and general anesthesia during surgery, serve to dissolve the interhemispheric connections and are, therefore, more conducive to autoscopic experiences. Grotstein cites the work of Gazzaniga and LeDoux (1978), which points to the possibility that each normal human being has one personality associated with a dominant hemisphere and another separate personality connected with a nondominant hemisphere. In ordinary daily life, the dominant hemisphere serves as a kind of "image rectifier," which fuses this dual consciousness and allows us to perceive events as a single consciousness.

3. Beyond interhemispheric split, Grotstein suggests, borrowing from the work of Katan (1954) and Bion (1957), that autoscopic experiences may reflect a dissociation between the psychotic and the nonpsychotic portions of the personality. Grotstein postulates a dual track of mental existence from the time of birth in which there is immediate postnatal separateness on one track while on another there is a continuation of primary identification with the mother. He speculates that autoscopic phenomena may be a manifestation of a

breech or discrepancy between the two tracks related to a defective object of primary identification, that is, the mothering figure. He connects this with a premature rupture of the sense of symbiosis with mother due to overstimulation, which he says may precipitate a precocious "two-ness." He says this pattern is typical of states of dissociation, and he believes that by virtue of its being a dissociative phenomenon, autoscopy should, therefore, be characterized as a special form of depersonalization.

4. As may be evident from the foregoing determinants, Grotstein views autoscopy as a regression. Specifically, he suggests that autoscopic experiences are representative of imagery emerging at the sensory threshold of the developmental period where the infant begins to experience mind-body separation. At the same developmental stage, according to Tausk (1919), the ego ideal is split-off and projected outward. Hence, the ego ideal may be a forerunner of the alter ago, other self, or imaginary companion. As Grotstein puts it, "The splitting off from the projection of the ego ideal makes a ladder available for a fantasied scaffold for the experience of a twin self, whether mentally or perceptually, as in autoscopic phenomena" (1983, p. 300). Grotstein says all of his case examples seem to experience their autoscopic double as uncanny, eerie, and yet strangely friendly. There is some sense of reexperiencing a lost and disavowed part of the self which has "returned home." The strange, but friendly, feeling about the double is characteristic, he says, and he asserts that autoscopic phenomena may be akin to transitional phenomena in which twin consciousnesses are sufficiently separate so that two different aspects of one's self can view one another.

While Grotstein's formulation of autoscopic phenomena is by far the most sophisticated and thoroughgoing in the literature, its very scope and breadth create certain difficulties in applying the formulation to clinical data. In his attempt to encompass a wide variety of normal and pathological forms of altered mind/body perception within a unifying scheme, he has blurred the distinctions between a number of different human experiences. His theoretical formulation is persuasive and undoubtedly applies to many altered states of consciousness. However, certain discrepancies are problematic. For example some autoscopic subjects do not have a friendly response to their doubles. As Lukianowicz (1958) points out, sadness or bewilderment are more common responses. Others, like Freud, may respond with revulsion. In fact there is a tendency in the literary use of the double as well as in clinical reports for the affective responses to fall into two general categories, that is, favorable and unfavorable. The double may be greeted with friendly admiration as a carbon copy of oneself and hence a narcissistic mirroring response, or, alternatively, may be greeted with revulsion and disgust as a disavowed part of the self returning from repression. It may well be that the extent to which projective identification is operating in any one particular case determines the reaction of the subject. For instance, if the double is a disavowed and unacceptable part of the self, that is, a container for all the "bad" parts of the psyche, its return may be seen as a failure of the defensive effort to externalize the "bad" and it may then regarded with contempt. The story of Dr. Jekyll and Mr. Hyde, where the self has been split into good and bad parts is an example of this motif. In cases where projective identification is not a prominent defensive determinant of the autoscopic double, the phantom may be much more welcome, as it does not represent a disavowed and unacceptable part of oneself. Moreover, although there may be similarities in the underlying mechanisms of autoscopy, depersonalization, and out-of-body experience, there are phenomenological and contextual differences, which, we would argue, should be preserved because they inform the clinician's choice of therapeutic intervention. For this reason in our efforts to differentiate out-of-body experience and autoscopy, we will preserve the narrow, clinical definition used by Lukianowicz (1958).

AUTOSCOPY VERSUS OBE

Since persons in the midst of out-of-body experiences are likely to see their bodies before them, there has been some tendency in the literature to confuse autoscopic phenomena and out-of-body experience. Lunn (1970), for example, reports three cases, which he refers to as autoscopic phenomena, but two of the three cases are classical out-of-body experiences. Sabom (1982) labels the out-of-body experience aspect of near-death experiences as "autoscopic near-death experiences." This confusion in the literature is all the more reason that we favor a narrower definition of autoscopy. Technically, autoscopic phenomena may not be a true form of altered mind/body perception since the mind remains identified with the body. Subjects do not think they are seeing their true bodies; rather, they have insight into the fact that they are seeing a phantom of themselves. The

Table 4.1
COMPARISON OF AUTOSCOPIC AND OBE

Autoscopic Phenomena	OBE
Mind remains identified with body and perceptual point of view is not altered.	Mind and point of perception are experienced as outside of body.
Subject sees apparitional "double" of himself.	Subject sees his own physical body.
"Double" is active and often imitates all movements.	"Double" is inactive.
Only face and shoulders are typically seen.	Whole body is seen.
Body often appears colorless and transparent.	Body appears real and lifelike.
Most frequent affect is sadness.	Sadness rare.
"Double" moves towards and away from observer.	"Double" is stationary while observing self moves.

subject's mind and body remain identified with one another, unlike the situation in an out-of-body experience. In other words the perceptual point of view is not altered. In an out-of-body experience, on the other hand, the mind is experienced as having shifted to an outside point in space from where it recognizes the physical body as real rather than as an image. This difference is the first important point in differentiating the two phenomena (see Table 4.1). Green (1968) recognizes this distinction and suggests that a more accurate term for the autoscopic experience would be "autophany," which means "to appear to oneself" rather than to see one's self. Autoscopy is actually a more accurate description of what we here are referring to as out-of-body experience since subjects believe that they are literally viewing themselves rather than an image that has appeared before them. However, to change the terminology at this point might simply lead to further confusion, so we will continue to use the more accepted terms.

Another distinction is that the autoscopic double is usually quite active when it appears to the subject, while the physical body appears in a restful and relaxed state to the person having an out-of-body experience. Lukianowicz also notes that most frequently the subject having an autoscopic hallucination sees only the face or the face and shoulders of the double, only infrequently seeing the entire body of the double. In contrast the person having an out-of-body experience, typically sees the entire body. Another differential point is that autosopic phenomena are usually characterized by a transparent, colorless double, whereas in OBE the body is perceived as lifelike. It is quite common for the autoscopic double to imitate all of the movements of the subject, particularly the facial expression, presenting a mirrorlike effect. In OBE the physical body is ordinarily motionless and at rest. The most frequent affect connected with autoscopic phenomena is sadness, according to Lukianowicz. As we have indicated, among the effects associated with OBEs, sadness is quite rare. Ostow (1960) points out that the observer in autoscopic experiences is stationary and the double moves toward or away from him. In out-of-body experience the "double," that is, the actual physical body, is stationary and the observer in the out-of-body state moves toward or away from it.

TREATMENT

Lukianowicz (1958) states that no treatment is known for primary idiopathic autoscopy. If the autoscopic phenomena are secondary to an organic lesion or a coexisting psychiatric disorder, treatment of the primary disorder is indicated. The migraine sufferer or the epileptic who has autoscopic experiences may well get relief from both the primary and the secondary autoscopy when the primary disorder is successfully treated. If autoscopy accompanies schizophrenia or depression, treatment of those entities may improve the autoscopy. Faguet (1979) emphasizes the importance of tending to the needs of the hospitalized patient to minimize the stresses of hospitalization as a prophylactic measure against autoscopic and other stress-related phenomena. Grotstein (1983) implies that to the extent that these phenomena represent failures of integration of parts of one's self, the autoscopic experiences will decrease or vanish as one integrates disparate views of one's self in the process of analytic working through of the paranoid-schizoid position and the depressive position. Little is actually known about the treatment of autoscopic phenomena, which reflects the inherent mystery of this bizarre syndrome and underscores the fact that this phantom, like most others, is elusive.

Five —— SCHIZOPHRENIC BODY BOUNDARY DISTURBANCES

Schizophrenia is a protean psychosis, manifesting a variety of disturbances in perception, cognition, affect, and behavior. Among these are distortions of the body image, particularly of the boundary that separates one's skin from the external environment. These difficulties in sorting out inner experience from external reality are obviously linked in an intimate way to generalized problems with reality testing. In fact Freeman et al. (1958) conclude that dissolution of ego boundaries is the basic disturbance in schizophrenia and that all other manifestations of the illness can be viewed as elaborations of this fundamental disturbance.

An examination of the bodily distortions of schizophrenics is relevant to our exploration of the field of altered mind/body perception for several reasons: careful study of highly pathological aberrations in the course of ego development provides expanded insight into the normal development of the body image and of the establishment of boundaries between one's self and the outside world; because of poorly established body boundaries, the schizophrenic patient often feels "out of the body," and his or her subjective reports may be confused with the out-of-body experience of the psychologically healthy individual; and skeptics may dismiss the out-of-body experience as merely the delusion or hallucination of a psychotic individual, so that it is important to delineate the significant differences between the body boundary disturbances of the schizophrenic individual and the OBE of the nondisturbed person. After reviewing, from a descriptive standpoint, the major clinical symptomatology involving bodily distortions in schizophrenic patients, we will discuss the developmental and theoretical considerations stemming from the clinical observations. To illustrate further the manner in which these distortions may present themselves in clinical practice, we will provide several case examples. The differentiation of the typical out-of-body experience from schizophrenic body boundary disturbances will then be discussed, followed by a short comment on the treatment of body image disturbances in schizophrenics.

CLINICAL MANIFESTATIONS OF BODY BOUNDARY DISTURBANCES

Body image disturbances, both in normal individuals and psychiatric patients, are probably much more common than is usually thought. Lukianowicz (1967), in a survey of body image disturbances among psychiatric inpatients, suggests that roughly one-fourth of all psychiatric patients experience some kind of disturbance of the body image, based on his study of 200 unselected consecutive admissions to Barrow Hospital in Bristol, England. Angyal (1935) found that 15 percent of 100 schizophrenics complained of body image disorders of various kinds. Lancaster (1954) studied 41 schizophrenic patients, and found that 31 percent complained of various somatic disturbances. Of Lukianowicz's sample of schizophrenic inpatients with body image disturbances, 61 percent experienced changes in the shape of their body image, 17 percent in its size, and 22 percent experienced a change in the position of their bodies in space. Body image disturbances were in no way correlated with demographic factors such as sex, age, education, intelligence, or social class.

There is certainly little question that schizophrenics are far more likely than neurotics or normals to display aberrations of body boundaries. Shukla (1972) studied 60 neurotics, 100 normal subjects, and 100 schizophrenics, matched for age, education, and socioeconomic status. Using the Holtzman Inkblot Technique to study their perception of body image boundaries, he demonstrated in a statistically significant manner that schizophrenics are much more likely than normals or neurotics to perceive their body image boundaries as diffuse and fragile. Normals and neurotics, on the other hand, showed no significant differences.

A variety of studies have sought to pinpoint a characteristic disturbance of body boundaries in the schizophrenic population, but the data available do not support the idea of a single, specifically schizophrenic pattern. On the contrary, the studies indicate that several different forms of bodily distortion are common. From our reading of the literature and our clinical experience, we are able to classify the body boundary disturbances of schizophrenics into seven general categories:

1. fusion phenomena;
2. the experience of one's body boundaries as fluid and constantly changing;
3. underestimation of one's own body size;
4. omission of hands and feet as part of the body image;
5. overestimation and underestimation of the size of body parts;
6. the feeling that one's body is not one's own (akin to depersonalization);
7. the feeling that one's body is unreal or a machine.

In this chapter we will focus primarily on the first five since we have considered depersonalization in Chapter Three, where we pointed out that it is a phenomenon that cuts across all diagnostic categories. Also, the experience of one's body as a machine, or otherwise unreal, is a fascinating symptom, but it is more of a somatic delusion than a form of altered mind/body perception involving misperception of body boundaries.

Various researchers have asked the schizophrenic patient to estimate the size of his body parts. The findings of these investigations are contradictory. Cleveland (1960) and Burton and Adkins (1961) found that schizophrenics tend to overestimate the size of their body parts. Weckowicz and Sommer (1960) found that schizophrenics underestimate the sizes of their hands and feet. Fisher and Seidner (1963) also found that in comparison to normals and neurotics, schizophrenics tend to perceive their body parts as decreased in size. Dillon (1962) found no differences between schizophrenics and controls in accuracy of estimating the size of their various body parts. In a later study Fisher (1966) compared schizophrenic patients to controls on several estimates of body-part size and found primarily nonsignificant differences. No simple answer presents itself to explain the contradiction.

Papson and Hamersma (1974) used slides of parental figures to assess how 20 male schizophrenics view their own size relative to a parental figure. Compared to a group of 20 normal males, these schizophrenics consistently underestimated their own body heights. They also tended more than normals did to overestimate the height of a maternal figure while underestimating the size of a paternal figure. Papson and Hamersma relate this to the theory of Lidz (Lidz et al. 1965) that families of schizophrenics are "skewed" in the direction of a dominant maternal figure, while the father is usually only peripherally involved with the child.

Kokonis (1972) administered the Draw-A-Person Test to 128 hospitalized schizophrenics and 104 normally functioning adult males. The results clearly indicated that a significantly greater number of schizophrenics, as compared to normal subjects, failed to depict hands, arms, feet, and legs in their drawings of a person. Their findings support the theoretical views of Schilder (1935) and Federn (1952) that there is a serious impairment of the cathexis of ego boundaries in the schizophrenic patient. According to this point of view, schizophrenics experience a narrowing of the body boundary in which the distal parts of the body are less ego-involved, and therefore are less cathected than the more proximal parts.

Some of the most sophisticated and detailed work in the area of boundary disturbances in schizophrenia has been that based on Rorschach responses. The perception of the boundaries of the inkblot seems to reflect the patient's intrapsychic boundary experiences. Fisher and Cleveland (1968) proposed the scoring of the patient's responses according to "barrier" and "penetration." The former indicates the extent to which boundedness is noted, while the latter reflects breakdown or fluidity of boundaries. As one would expect, schizophrenic patients have been observed to make a much higher number of penetration responses and a much lower number of barrier responses as compared to neurotics and normals (Holtzman et al. 1961). Two other types of responses that have been studied in psychiatric patients are contamination and fabulized combination. Contamination involves the combining of two normally separated percepts into one incongruous percept, while fabulized combination is defined as the arbitrary or incongruous combination of two percepts while the separateness of the two components is maintained.

Quinlan and Harrow (1974) studied 171 psychiatric inpatients according to their Rorschach responses and scored the relative frequencies of these four response areas in comparison to diagnostic categories. They found that schizophrenics have significantly more contamination responses than any other group of disturbed patients.

Fabulized combinations are more frequent in schizophrenics and latent schizophrenics than in depressive patients. However, no significant differences were found for barrier percentage scores. Moreover, penetration responses were not reliably linked to schizophrenics, indicating that barrier and penetration responses are not pathognomonic for schizophrenia. However, the study of Quinlan and Harrow certainly confirms that schizophrenics give certain specific types of responses, that is, contamination responses, on the Rorschach that are indicative of profound boundary disturbances.

Traub et al. (1967) used a distorting mirror in their studies of normals and schizophrenics to allow the subject to adjust the mirror until the subject felt that an accurate perception of himself or herself was perceived in the mirror. Schizophrenics were consistently less accurate in their perception of their bodies. However, they also distorted a rectangular frame and allowed the schizophrenic subjects to adjust the mirror until the frame was accurately reflected. They conclude that the disturbance of body image in schizophrenia is part of a more general visual-perceptual disturbance that is part and parcel of the illness. Chapman et al. (1978) came to a similar conclusion. They constructed a 28 item true-false scale to measure schizophrenic body image aberration. They found that schizophrenics have significantly more body image aberration than normal controls. Fourteen of 28 items were particularly useful in distinguishing the two groups—these included items that dealt with the body seeming dead or unreal, decayed, misshapen, smaller than usual, not one's own, seeming to melt into surroundings, being indistinguishable from other objects, seeming to remain attached to objects touched, taking on the appearance of another person's body, and incorporating external objects. The authors also included some items on perceptual aberrations that do not involve the body image, such as perception of furniture or other neutral objects in the environment. The schizophrenics who were deviant in their body image scores were also deviant in their perception of other items in their environment. Hence, they conclude that the body image aberration of schizophrenia appears to be an aspect of a broader perceptual problem.

A DEVELOPMENTAL UNDERSTANDING

To understand these multivaried disturbances catalogued previously, we now turn to a developmental perspective. The bizarre alterations of mind/body perception described previously have challenged the minds of clinical observers for many years. One of the earliest contributions to the understanding of these phenomena in schizophrenics was the seminal paper by Tausk, "Origin of the Influencing Machine in Schizophrenia" (1919). In this essay Tausk brilliantly explains the development of a schizophrenic's delusion that an external machine was influencing his behavior by tracing it to a change in bodily sensation in the patient, which he in turn relates to a regression to a developmental phase when bodily sensations were experienced as unacceptable and alien. Hence, Tausk understands the delusion as a regressive projection of the patient's own body into the external environment. In this context he coined the concept, "ego boundary." He asserted that very early bodily experiences of the infant were critical in the establishment and maintenance of the normal ego boundary. If, for some reason, the body cathexis is disturbed during early infantile development, the ego boundaries become prone to disintegration, Tausk theorized.

The ego is the center of mature intraphysic functioning, and the impairments of ego functioning in schizophrenia have caught the attention of all clinicians who have studied the illness. Ego functions such as reality testing, object relations, judgment, autonomous functioning, and mastery of one's environment are frequently impaired to a devastating degree in schizophrenia. Many investigators have felt that the ego deficiencies of schizophrenia are intimately related to faulty formation of body boundaries. Freud noted, in 1923, that "the ego is first and foremost a bodily ego; it is not merely a surface entity, but it is itself a projection of a surface" (p. 26). In 1927 Freud added a footnote to this discussion: "The ego is ultimately derived from bodily sensations, chiefly from those springing from the surface of the body. It may thus be regarded as a mental projection from the surface of the body" (p. 26). Hence, Freud implied that the development of one's body image was instrumental to the development of competent psychological functioning and, by implication, to the pathogenetic aberration of the schizophrenic patient.

Federn (1952) further developed this notion with his far-reaching formulations on the importance of ego cathexis. Whereas other writers had emphasized the withdrawal of object cathexis into an autistic shell in schizophrenia, Federn emphasized the withdrawal of ego boundary cathexis. He notes that in every case of schizophrenia, the ego boundary can no longer be psychologically invested by the patient, and a dissolution of the barrier between what is inside and what is outside occurs. Federn writes that this impairment of ego boundaries is not simply a symptom of the illness, but it is in fact the basic process during the whole course of the illness.

In her study of childhood psychosis, Mahler (1952) focused on the importance of the mother-infant dyad in the development of the body image. Only through the rhythmic fondling, cuddling, and other varieties of bodily contact with the mother, says Mahler, can the infant differentiate a firm sense of his body ego out of the boundaryless state with mother. She points out that every infant begins life in an undifferentiated state where the mother's body parts are viewed as part of one's self. Mahler hypothesizes that in the absence of the normal somatosensory stimulation in the mother-infant dyad, the infant cannot develop a sense of his own body integrity, leading to profound distortions in every aspect of later ego development, as well as the cognitive and perceptual disturbances typical of schizophrenia. Mahler's conceptualization allows us to understand the emergence of body boundary disturbances in the adult schizophrenia as regressive reactivations of early sensations of being merged or fused with one's mother. While these episodes may be experienced as disintegrating, they also may provide some defensive or wish-fulfilling function in that they recapture the symbiotic bliss of the earliest months of life. This combination of the effort to recapture the "paradise lost" of infancy and the dread of catastrophic annihilation forms an overwhelming and paradoxical dilemma for the schizophrenic, that is, the regression to the oceanic state of oneness with mother requires a dissolution of the body ego. The schizophrenic is drawn magnetically to this state, while at the same time dreading it.

Blatt and Wild (1976) have devoted an entire monograph to the thesis that the broad variety of symptoms associated with schizophrenia can all be understood as later manifestations of early developmental disturbances in the capacity to experience, perceive, and represent boundaries. Their specific focus is on the boundary between self and object, and they draw on both the theories of developmental psychology and the psychoanalytic formulations of object relations theory to support their central idea. They assert that the level of boundary disturbance is very much related to the degree of disruption in early object relationships. Those patients whose body boundaries are most impaired seem to be those with the most extensive chaos in early relationships. Hence, schizophrenic patients with more minimal boundary disturbances tend to have had more adequate past relationships. They suggest that the degree of boundary disruption provides a quantifiable variable for differentiating the severity of schizophrenia. Those schizophrenics with the most difficulty in articulating boundaries tend to be the most disturbed chronic patients, who have a history of impoverished object relations and a very poor prognosis. They share Mahler's view that the nature and quality of the early infant-mother relationship affects the capacity for cognitive differentiation and the establishment of clear self-objects boundaries. They also emphasize that the establishment of boundaries is fundamental to the accurate perception of the object, that is, other persons in the environment.

Grand (1982) has carefully studied the developmental problems of schizophrenics, and he believes that the peculiarities in sensation, perception, orientation, and motor behavior are all related to a generalized failure to integrate very early body experiences, which would otherwise contribute to the development of a cohesive body self. This early disturbance in the development of the body ego, in his opinion, constitutes the core of the mental disturbances in schizophrenia. Citing the research of others, as well as his own, he suggests that the integration of somatosensory and vestibular sensory input is absolutely essential to perceptual-motor and cognitive growth. Specifically, self-initiated somatosensory feedback seems to be crucial. Grand says that it is the child's recognition of himself or herself as the initiator of action that ultimately helps him or her to distinguish between self and object. If the infant does not become adequately aware of his or her own role in generating both pleasurable and unpleasurable stimulation to his or her body, a profound disturbance in body ego formation ensues. Grand has made the clinical observation that the schizophrenic patient who touches himself in the service of stimulation is actually attempting to bolster disintegrating boundaries between himself or herself and the world of objects. Grand provides a significant contribution to our clinical understanding of the schizophrenic patient in that he extends the notion that the patient's tendency to self-stimulate is only for the purposes of tension discharge. He makes it clear that such self-stimulating experience also maintains the integrity of the body ego and avoids the catastrophic dissolution or fragmentation of the ego. Grand's view is that self-experience and personal identity are also lacking in schizophrenics since there has never been a complete separation from the maternal figure. Hence, the patients never experience themselves as the initiator of their own actions and are chronically vulnerable to feeling symbiotically dependent on another person, who may leave them at any time and cause them to fragment.

The viewpoint expressed by Blatt and Wild, in addition to other authors mentioned previously, that the primary underlying disturbance in schizophrenia is related to faulty development of the body ego in the earliest developmental stages of life, is not only useful in explaining many of the peculiar distortions of the relationship between mind and body. It is also helpful in explaining apparently coincidental improvements in schizophrenic patients when they are suffering from a serious physical illness. Freeman et al. (1958) comment on the fact that clinicians have long observed that a schizophrenic patient, no matter how chronic, may seem suddenly better when a physical illness supercedes. They explain this curious finding on the basis of increased bodily sensations associated with the pain or discomfort of the illness, leading to an increase in the patient's cathexis of his body ego. The fact that the entirety of the schizophrenic symptomatology improves with an improvement in the accurate perception of the body ego (in association with increased cathexis) lends support to the idea that the disturbance of the body image is central to the illness.

At this point clinical examples may be helpful in further illustrating both the descriptive symptomatology and the underlying theoretical considerations involved in these disturbances.

CASE EXAMPLES

Miss G. was a 22-year-old, severely schizophrenic woman who was seen by one of the authors (G.O.G.) in intensive psychotherapy for a period of four years. She experienced a number of "fusion" phenomena during that time, manifested by repeatedly misidentifying in others attributes of herself and attributes of those around her in herself. One striking episode of this type occurred during a psychotic episode and serves as a particularly useful illustration since the patient misidentifies her experience as an out-of-body experience. In the patient's own words, "It was like an out-of-body experience. An identity problem. I was not in my body. I was in Jane's (another patient). No, she was in me. She was sitting in me. I don't know where I was. I couldn't locate myself. One thing for certain—I wasn't in my body."

Miss G. had particular problems differentiating herself from Jane. When Jane mutilated herself, Miss G. felt that she must also mutilate herself. Jane had once attempted to enucleate her right eye and had a residual strabismus. During another psychotic episode, Miss G. similarly attempted to enucleate her eye. In the psychotherapy she asked the therapist never to bring up Jane since she would begin to think that she must do the things that Jane did. The preceding quotation as well as the other historical material clearly represent instances of fusion, that is, Miss G. was unable to form a boundary between herself and the other patient in her environment. The experience is also clearly different from the typical out-of-body experience, and we will further differentiate these two entities later in the chapter.

Miss H. was a 33-year-old married woman with two children when she became pregnant for the third time. She had been diagnosed schizophrenic a number of years before and required a large amount of antipsychotic medication. Sixteen days following the birth of her third child, she nearly died from a postpartum hemorrhage connected with a failed tubal ligation. She was otherwise physically healthy. The stress of the hemorrhage caused the patient to begin to decompensate, so she was admitted to a psychiatric unit to stabilize her and to assist her with breast feeding. She was having a good deal of difficulty breast feeding because of delusional ideas about her breasts. She talked about the shape of her breasts continuously and was very anxious that they were no longer attractive to men. She said that sexual thoughts connected with her breasts kept her from feeding. She experienced the act of nursing as though the baby were stretching her nipple like gum until it fell off. She was convinced that when the nipple fell off, she would not longer be sexually attractive.

As this patient became increasingly psychotic, she was placed in seclusion. While in seclusion with the baby, the nursing staff found her trying to stuff the baby into her vagina. When questioned by the staff as to why she was attempting to return the baby to the womb, she said that her vagina was so enormous that she could accommodate the baby as well as various items of furniture, such as chairs and tables. While in seclusion, she was unable to distinguish herself from a pool of feces on the seclusion room floor. She asked the nursing staff, "Why aren't you cleaning me up?" Fortunately, the patient responded to increasing doses of thiothixene and lithium, and her psychotic symptoms, along with the body image distortions, went into remission. Another relevant detail in this patient's history is that she was completely unable to separate from her own mother. Her psychiatrist noted that he was never clear whether she were talking about herself or her mother. A persistent symbiotic relationship between her own mother and her made it only seem natural to attempt to return her baby to the state of oneness of the in utero existence.

Mr. I. was a 20-year-old single male college student who was admitted to the hospital with persecutory delusions involving his conviction that he was the victim of intense harrassment by students in the dormitory and that he was being terrorized by a conspiracy of rejection in his own family. He said the students in his dormitory ridiculed him for being a "hippy" and teased him about having an erection that he felt they could see through the folds of his clothing. When he attempted to watch football games on television, he could hear students in the crowd harrassing him about his erections and about his inability to urinate in the presence of others. The patient felt this latter difficulty led to accusations by the students that he was a homosexual. Mr. I. was also a peculiar looking individual: he was quite short in stature, with marked scoliosis of the thoracic spine and shoulders that were so broad that they were out of proportion with the rest of his body. He also had a club foot. However, whatever the reality was regarding his actual appearance, he had grossly distorted perceptions of his own body. As he sat in meetings with his psychiatrist, he often imagined that the bones in his head were changing positions and lending a grotesque appearance to his face. He also experienced his muscles alternately growing and shrinking in his arms and legs. He had delusional ideas about his genitals, involving paresthesia-like sensations which he was convinced led to involuntary erections.

As with many paranoid schizophrenics, a severe problem with self-esteem was at the core of his illness. This issue became more and more prominent as he was able to open up more to his doctor. He felt he was unspeakably ugly and deformed, and he felt sexually inadequate to a marked degree. The fluidity of his body contours thus served an important purpose in his psychic equilibrium. It was preferable for him to think that his muscles and bones were constantly growing and shifting than to face the reality that he was imprisoned permanently inside an impaired, misshapened body. Similarly, the delusions about his genitals and his involuntary erections served as a defense against his feelings of impotence and sexual unattractiveness. The patient made dramatic improvements with psychotherapy and antipsychotic medication. As his psychotic symptoms went into remission, his body distortions also disappeared.

Mr. J. was a chronic hebephrenic schizophrenic who was grossly disorganized in behavior, cognition, and affective expression. His appearance was bizarre and at times humorous because of his tendency to wear several pairs of pants at one time. He was convinced that his body was so large that he had to wear several pairs of pants to adequately cover it. Lukianowicz (1967) notes that the body image commonly encompasses clothes as well as the body itself and, hence, is not restricted by the boundary of the skin. One might speculate in the case of Mr. J. that one or more pairs of trousers may have been incorporated into his body image so that when he put on the third or fourth pair, he felt he was putting on his first.

SCHIZOPHRENIC BODY BOUNDARY DISTURBANCES VERSUS OBE

As mentioned previously, the loss of body boundaries involved in the illness of schizophrenia may be confused with an out-of-body experience, as was the case with Miss G. Alternatively, an out-of-body experience may be regarded by some as a psychotic episode involving body boundary disturbances. The experiences are actually quite different, and there are several points of differential diagnosis that one can use to delineate the schizophrenic experience from that of a person having an out-of-body experience (see Table 5.1). First, the hallmark of schizophrenia is psychosis—that is, loss of reality testing. As Lukianowicz (1967) points out, schizophrenic body image disturbances are often accompanied by hallucinations of smell, hearing, or vision, by ideas of reference, and by frank delusions. During or after the experience, the schizophrenic is likely to form a delusional elaboration of the experience. In persons having an out-of-body experience, on the other hand, reality testing remains intact. As we demonstrated in Chapter Two, subjects reporting out-of-body experiences tend to be free from any signs of mental illness. In fact our sample appears to be psychologically healthier than controls. Another important distinction is that the schizophrenic who has perceptual disturbances concerning his or her body is often chronically plagued with those disturbances, whereas those experiencing OBE have episodic and short-lived alterations in body boundaries.

As we have demonstrated in this chapter, the bodily distortions of schizophrenics are highly varied. As Lukianowicz (1967) illustrates with his statistics, distortions of shape are by far the most prevalent body image disturbances, comprising 61 percent of his

Table 5.1
COMPARISON OF SCHIZOPHRENIC LOSS OF BODY BOUNDARIES AND OBE

Schizophrenic Loss of Body Boundaries	OBE
Loss of reality testing.	Reality testing intact.
Chronic difficulty with delineation of body boundaries.	Episodic and short-lived.
Bodily distortions varied.	Distortion basically unvaried.
Location of body is often uncertain.	Location of body is clear.
Profound regression of personality.	No evidence of regression.
Identity is lost and blurred with others—an experience of dissolution.	Identity intact—an integrating experience.
Experienced as "going crazy."	Not experienced as "going crazy."

schizophrenic sample, while only 17 percent have distortions of size, and a mere 22 percent distortions of position. Within these three categories the misperceptions are even further varied and may be highly idiosyncratic, as indicated by some of the case examples provided. By contrast the alteration in one's mind/body relationship in out-of-body experience is relatively unvaried and specific; indeed, the physical body itself, when viewed from the new point of perception, generally appears undistorted. Another differential point is the fact that schizophrenics are frequently uncertain as to the location of the body in space, as was the case with Miss G. during her fusion experience. The subject of an out-of-body experience, on the other hand, is usually much more certain about the location of his or her body. Most subjects report that it is in the immediate environment, sitting in a chair, lying on a bed, and so on.

Profound regression of the personality is typical of the schizophrenic patient during an episode of disintegration, since all ego functions seem to suffer as a result of fragmentation of the body. However, there is no evidence of such regression in the person having an OBE. Similarly, the schizophrenic's identity is lost and blurred with others when he or she has a fusion experience, producing a sense of dissolution. The person having an out-of-body experience retains his or her identity, often describing the experience as integrating and transforming in a positive sense rather than disorganizing. Whereas the schizophrenic patients are likely to feel that they are going crazy amidst the panic of disorientation about their bodies, persons having an OBE rarely feel that they are losing their minds. If the OBE is a regression, it is certainly a regression in the service of the ego rather than one in which the ego is overwhelmed and fragmented, such as in the schizophrenic's experience.

While these points of differential diagnosis are useful for the clinician, a caveat is indicated at this point. Schizophrenia is a psychiatric diagnosis; out-of-body experience is not. We have no reason to believe that the OBE is restricted to certain nosologic categories in psychiatry, nor can we assert that it only occurs in normals. It is certainly possible that a schizophrenic patient could have an out-of-body experience, as we have defined it, quite apart from other episodes of body boundary disturbance. The impaired ego of the schizophrenic might find such an experience difficult to integrate, and it might be delusionally elaborated. This possibility raises important theoretical and conceptual questions, which we will address more fully in Chapter Eleven.

TREATMENT

Since the 1950s, antipsychotic medication has been the cornerstone of the treatment of schizophrenia. Whether the body image disturbances of schizophrenics are responsive to antipsychotic medication, however, is highly controversial. Both Cardone and Olson (1969) and Jenkins and Sambroski (1964) report that antipsychotic medication does not alter the bodily distortions of chronic schizophrenics. Freedman et al. (1965) report that these disturbances are indeed responsive to thiothixene treatment. Lukianowicz (1967) asserts that in his sample of schizophrenic patients, the body image disturbances disappeared simultaneously with the acute psychotic symptoms when the patients were treated along conventional lines for their psychiatric illness per se, with no special attention given to the body image disturbances. In other words the usual dosages of antipsychotic medication designed to treat schizophrenia are adequate therapeutic interventions for the body image disturbance. One can only speculate on the reasons for these discrepancies. The level of chronicity of the patient in question may be involved, and, of course, one must wonder about compliance, dosage levels, active blood and tissue levels, and duration of treatment in each case.

Some researchers have sought to improve the bodily aberrations of the schizophrenic patients through informed application of the understanding of the body boundary disturbances inherent in the illness. Goertzel (1965) applied the body ego technique (BET) to 36 chronic, regressed schizophrenic patients. This approach involves focusing attention on body posture and movement as they relate to body image, on the patient's sense of time as experienced with different speeds of movement, on body ego boundaries, and on reality contact and experience in movement. It amounts to a deliberate attempt to recreate for the schizophrenic patient the physical experience of the postures and movements associated with a wide range of emotions and attitudes. In their study those patients treated with BET did significantly better than controls in terms of overall improvement, affective contacts, and nursing ratings of motility and general functioning. Darby (1970) used similar somatic awareness techniques with a group of chronic schizophrenic inpatients. He used barrier and penetration scores on Inkblot responses prior to the somatic awareness technique and after the sessions had been completed. Highly significant increases in the barrier score from pretest to posttest were achieved by those patients who experienced actual physical stimulation, while those who did not, the control group, remained the same. Penetration scores, on the other hand, were unaffected by the experimental manipulations. The treatment of schizophrenia, in general, is embroiled in controversy regarding the need for hospitalization, the length of stay, the use of antipsychotic medications, the use of anti-Parkinson medications, and the benefits of psychotherapy. The controversy over whether or not body boundary disturbances are influenced by various forms of therapy is only a microcosm of the greater debate over the most effective form of treatment of schizophrenia.

In Chapters Three, Four, and Five, we have covered the major forms of altered mind/body perception that are likely to be confused with out-of-body experience. We are aware, however, that still other clinical entities exist. Although drug use was quite limited among the subjects of our study, the literature reports "floating" states very similar to out-of-body experience in persons under the influence of certain drugs. Lukianowicz (1967) reports these experiences in two patients treated with haloperidol and in one patient treated with alpha-methyl-dopa. As early as 1859, Mantegazza gave an account of cocaine intoxication during which he felt he was floating through the air out of his body amid colorful visions. Hallucinogens such as LSD and mescaline have produced a wide variety of bodily distortions, and these experiences may or may not be similar to those of persons reporting out-of-body experiences.

We will now turn to an examination of normal altered states of consciousness and seek to differentiate these experiences from the out-of-body experience.

Six — "MORE REAL THAN A DREAM"

Prudentius (348-420 B.C.), in a charm against nightmares, says, "Be far, oh far from us, you monsters of our disordered dreams! Be far from us, demon, with your subtle deceptions! Depart, oh tortuous serpent, who with a thousand quarrels and subtle frauds agitates our peaceful hearts!" There isn't a person alive who has not at some time had a nightmare. The terrifying nightmare is clearly not part of our ordinary reality, and we never stop to think about making that differentiation. The closer the dream experience comes to waking life, the more difficult it is to distinguish from reality. Dreams are often like landscapes. When one wakes up, they are all around one, and one has to move a certain distance away from them to see what they are.

At this point we will deal with the problem posed by the many subjects (94 percent) in our study, who stated most emphatically that the experience they had was "more real than a dream," that is, not a dream at all. The strength of this assertion is highlighted by the interesting fact that at the time of the out-of-body experience, 36 percent (117 subjects) of the subjects said that they were dreaming, of which 97 Ss (83 percent) said the dream involved flying or falling. One implication of this finding is that the subjects themselves were able to discriminate clearly between dreaming and the out-of-body state and between dreaming and "waking reality." One possible interpretation of the out-of-body experience is that it is a form of a rapid eye movement (REM) dream, a daydream, or a manifestation of psychiatric disease. In Chapters Three, Four, and Five, we considered its differentiation from psychiatric syndromes. In this chapter we will distinguish the state from some commonly occurring altered states of consciousness, specifically, the lucid dream, the night dream, the daydream, and the twilight hypnagogic and hypnopompic states. We will also make comments on variations within these states of reverie: the Isakower phenomenon and the special cases of flying and falling dreams.

Let us begin with an example. Mrs. K., a 35-year-old mother of three children who has been the subject of intensive individual study in our research, and who has had out-of-body experiences and other unusual alterations in consciousness since the age of ten, was asked the following question: How do you know that the out-of-body state is not a dream? She replied: "I know the difference between a dream and the waking state...and the waking state is that in which I find myself during the OBE, though this level of awareness varies from time to time. I have experienced many different 'degrees' of consciousness during the OBE, but I've found that I am able to differentiate between even the 'fuzziest' of OBEs and a dream. I 'know' this in the same sense that I know that I'm drinking a cup of coffee as I type these words."

This experienced subject clearly considers the question a silly one and considers its answer self-evident. In her answer Mrs. K. illustrates many of the important assumptions made about physical waking reality. For example an integrated sense of one's body is absent in a dream, but present in the out-of-body state. In fact as Dr. L., a 40-year-old research scientist recorded, "I had been trying out these audio tapes that were supposed to induce an out-of-body experience and suddenly found myself standing beside the recliner I had been lying on. I could hear the tape playing through the stereo headphones and assumed I had gone to sleep and jerked myself awake. I turned to walk back to the recliner and was shocked by the sight of a body lying there, which I soon recognized as my own. It was not until I saw this recognizable physical body, that I realized that I was in any state other than that of being fully awake."

These examples serve to illustrate that the observing and experiencing parts of the self are integrated into one state in the OBE, as emphasized in Chapter Three. In a dream one does not dream about being in one's bedroom looking at one's body, as is common in the out-of-body state. In a dream the dreamer feels, "I am my body." It is not common to even see oneself in a dream. One is usually the invisible "camera operator."*

Mrs. M., a 37-year-old housewife described how she distinguished the out-of-body experience from a dream and from the waking state in a dramatic account of what she felt was "losing control over my OBEs." She says, "The main reason I prevented further OBEs from occurring was because of one experience in which I somehow lost control over them. I returned to my body one night,† and I decided to wake up. After doing so, I was terrified to find that my entire bedroom and bed were on fire! Later on, presumably on waking, I discovered that instead of going back into my physical body and awakening as I normally did, I somehow had lost control and had gone into a dream state." The considerable ease in controlling the out-of-body experience is not characteristic of normal night dreams, but is characteristic of the lucid dream, about which we will have more to say later.

THE OBE WITHIN A DREAM

What then does our data say about the OBE within a dream? In our study of 339 subjects, summarized in Tables 6.1 and 6.2, we find information about the differences between the OBE that occurs while dreaming, more specifically, within a flying or falling dream, on the one hand, and other out-of-body experiences and near-death experiences, on the other.

OBE dreamers tended to be people who had had more than one out-of-body experience. In Chapter One we noted that subjects who were in the top 25 percent in terms of the number of out-of-body experiences tended to have more vivid features, including a number of those listed for the dream OBE and the NDE. However, statistical examination of the data using univariate group independent t-tests failed to find that the dream OBEs were significantly more frequently represented in the top 25 percent of subjects, suggesting that the

---

*The exception is the occasional depersonalization dream, where, at a distance, one watches oneself participate in the action of the dream.

†This is often described in a disarmingly flippant manner by experienced out-of-body "travellers."

Table 6.1
THE DREAM OBE

Independent variable: At time of OBE were you dreaming?
1=Yes 2=No

Dependent Variables		X	S.D.	t	dF	P
Have you had more than one OBE?						
	Yes	1.174	0.381	−4.79	287	0.0001
	No	1.410	0.493			
During OBE did you feel sadness?						
	Yes	1.767	0.425	*−3.82	293	0.0001
	No	1.923	0.269			
Freedom.	Yes	1.254	0.438	*−1.99	305	0.047
	No	1.365	0.483			
Sense of energy.	Yes	1.360	0.482	*−264	309	0.009
	No	1.515	0.501			
During early stage did you hear music or singing?						
	Yes	1.760	0.430	*−2.22	195	0.028
	No	1.881	0.325			
Did you see a brilliant light which seemed to be a being of some kind?						
	Yes	1.571	0.500	*−2.58	165	0.011
	No	1.760	0.429			
Were you in the same environment as your physical body?						
	Yes	1.472	0.502	* 2.80	307	0.013
	No	1.328	0.471			
Were you aware of beings who acted as guides, helpers or teachers?						
	Yes	1.676	0.470	*−2.26	310	0.024
	No	1.791	0.408			

Dependent Variables	X	S.D.	t	dF	P
Looking back on it, is it something you want to try again?					
Yes	1.048	0.214	*−2.56	305	0.011
No	1.144	0.352			
Was it like traveling to a far off land?					
Yes	1.350	0.479	*−3.27	303	0.001
No	1.545	0.499			
Age of *First* OBE. (years)					
Yes	24.981	15.219	*−.276	308	0.006
No	29.769	14.071			
Absorption scale scores.					
Yes	25.077	6.833	* 3.46	317	0.001
No	21.858	8.540			

*Heterogeneous variance

Table 6.2
THE FLYING OR FALLING DREAM OBE

Independent variable: If you were dreaming, did the dreams involve flying or falling?
1=Yes   2=No

		X	S.D.	t	dF	P
Have you had more than one OBE?						
	Yes	1.117	0.323	−5.36	258	0.0001
	No	1.378	0.486			
During OBE did you feel:						
Joy	Yes	1.310	0.465	*−2.65	262	0.009
	No	1.480	0.501			
Sadness	Yes	1.765	0.427	*−3.53	257	0.001
	No	1.920	0.273			
Freedom	Yes	1.191	0.395	*−2.97	264	0.003
	No	1.367	0.483			
Power	Yes	1.595	0.494	*−2.33	257	0.021
	No	1.737	0.441			

Did you have a sense of energy?						
	Yes	1.292	0.457	*−3.34	268	0.001
	No	1.503	0.501			
In early stages did you hear music or singing?						
	Yes	1.727	0.450	*−2.64	174	0.009
	No	1.884	0.321			
Did you feel vibrations before or while leaving your body?						
	Yes	1.522	0.502	*−2.00	275	0.047
	No	1.647	0.479			
Were you in the same environment as your physical body?						
	Yes	1.471	0.054	* 2.45	255	0.015
	No	1.317	0.034			
Were you aware of other beings in non-physical form with you in OBE state?						
	Yes	1.506	0.503	*−3.46	274	0.001
	No	1.714	0.453			
Were you aware of beings who acted as guides, helpers or teachers for you?						
	Yes	1.615	0.489	*−4.18	268	0.0001
	No	1.838	0.370			
Did you see a brilliant light which seemed to be a being of some kind?						
	Yes	1.518	0.504	*−3.57	151	0.0001
	No	1.788	0.411			
Did you feel there was a purpose connected to the experience?						
	Yes	1.279	0.451	*−2.18	254	0.03
	No	1.418	0.495			

Dependent Variables	X	S.D.	t	dF	P
Looking back on the OBE was it:					
Something you want to try again?					
Yes	1.023	0.152	* 2.67	263	0.008
No	1.123	0.329			
An experience of great beauty?					
Yes	1.250	0.436	*−2.03	267	0.043
No	1.374	0.485			
Like traveling to a far off land?					
Yes	1.259	0.441	*−4.51	261	0.0001
No	1.545	0.499			
Reminiscent of childhood experiences?					
Yes	1.682	0.468	*−2.80	262	0.006
No	1.832	0.375			
Age of *First* OBE. (years)					
Yes	22.500	14.436	*−4.16	266	0.0001
No	30.140	13.965			
Absorption scale score.					
Yes	25.570	7.172	* 2.84	275	0.0005
No	22.755	8.067			

* Heterogenous variance.

increased numbers of OBEs. The experience itself is not usually in the same environment as the physical body, in contrast with the more typical OBE profile where the individual sees his or her own body from a vantage point of floating above it.

In Chapter Seven we describe the special variation of the out-of-body experience called the near-death experience. It seems as if the dreamers, particularly the flying and falling dreamers, have an out-of-body experience very similar to the near-death experience. Thus, the dream OBE is something that is quite attractive and pleasant to the individual, something they would want to try again, something that has a great sense of purpose, beauty, and, in the case of the flying and falling dream OBE, reminiscent of childhood experiences. In particular the OBE dreamer tends to have an experience less like physical reality than the "prototypical OBE" (see Chapter One).

Of the 117 subjects who were dreaming prior to having their out-of-body experience, only seven were near death at the time, of which five described their dream as flying or falling in type. The near-death experiencers had high absorption scores as did the OBE dreamers. This score, developed by Tellegen (1974), has been extensively used in research with altered states of consciousness as a measure of capacity to direct attention internally. The OBE dreamers and near-death experiencers share similarities in that they do tend to have a unique perceptual style.

Others working in this area, for example, Irwin (1980), have also noted similar perceptual-cognitive differences. As we reported in Chapter Two, Irwin found in a small, uncontrolled study of Australian out-of-body experiencers that they tended to be somewhat more neurotic and poor visualizers, an interesting finding in view of the tendency of the out-of-body experiencer to emphasize the bodily experience and the importance of movement through space, rather than the visual elements of the OBE. Thus, in one sense there seems to be more of the intrusion of the dreamlike, fantastic material into the out-of-body state, but the OBE subject who begins an OBE while dreaming is clearly able to distinguish the two states. Table 6.3 compares the near-death experience, the dream OBE, the prototypical OBE, and the flying or falling dream OBE.

The near-death experience and the out-of-body experience during a dream share at least one thing in common: the possibility that anoxic and/or toxic-metabolic stimuli may partially account for the phenomenology of the experience. Siegel (1980) has inferred something similar in an oft-quoted, controversial article on the near-death experience as an hallucinatory state. It is known that in the primate, in the cat, and possibly in the human being, during REM dreaming there can be considerable changes in blood pressure and a marked variability in the rate of respiration (Kramer 1969, p. 22). Hence, it might be reasonable to hypothesize a "normal" degree of anoxia in the brain during dream states.

THE REM DREAM

The psychophysiology of dreaming is complex and confused. Lewis Carroll appropriately described the state of affairs in *Alice's Adventures in Wonderland*: "The croquet balls were like hedgehogs, and the mallets live flamingos, and soldiers had to double

Table 6.3
A COMPARISON OF TYPES OF OBE

	NDE	Dream OBE	Flying Dream OBE	OBE Prototype
Heard sounds in early stages.	+	+	+	−
Tunnel.	+	−	−	−
Physical body visible.	+	−	−	+
Non-physical being present.	+	+	+	−
Brilliant light.	+	+	+	−
Vibrations.	−	−	+	−
Energy.	−	+	+	+
Highly positive experience.	+	+	+	+
Absorption Score.	Higher than controls	Higher than controls	Higher than controls	No difference
Age of 1st OBE.	28 yrs.	25 yrs.	23 yrs.	28 yrs.
Reminiscent of childhood experience.	−	−	+	−

+ = Present usually

− = Absent usually

themselves up and stand on their hands and feet to make the arches....Alice soon came to the conclusion that it was a difficult game indeed." In a detailed review of the literature of the mind in sleep, Arkin (1978) concludes that few findings with regard to the psychophysiology of sleep mentation have unequivocal agreement between different workers. Another problem in correlating physiology with dreaming is the problem of defining what a dream actually is. Vague definitions of dreaming have been used by experimenters in their attempts to communicate with their subjects. In one of the early studies by Aserinsky and Kleitman (1953), the definition of dreaming was simply "report detailed dreams," and for Pivik and Foulkes (1968), the presence of "some mentation" was regarded as a dream.

Others were more specific, such as Foulkes (1962), "any occurrence with visual, auditory, or kinesthetic imagery."

This situation has not changed a great deal. Researchers assume that the individual subject knows what a dream is. There are, however, specific physiological attributes. Phases of rapid eye movements occur as part of every 90-minute, sleep-dream cycle and are much more common during the latter part of the night. This REM phase is accompanied by motor paralysis and muscle tension with periodic intense outbursts of phasic activity. Other physiological concomitants are penile erection, decrease in brain temperature, irregular blood pressure and respiration, and low voltage, non-synchronized EEG activity, similar to the waking EEG (Snyder 1969).

No adequate physiological studies of the out-of-body state have been performed. In Chapter Twelve we describe an out-of-body experience in a naive subject that shows a most interesting EEG configuration, certainly unlike that seen in REM sleep. In the EEG studies of Miss Z. by Charles Tart (1968), in the studies of Blue Harary by Morris et al. (1978), and in our own studies of Monroe (Twemlow 1977), no unusual eye movements were noted. Tart's findings will be considered in more detail later; these include alphoid EEG with low amplitude similar to stage one sleep. In general the EEG data available on OBEs indicate that they do not occur during phases traditionally considered to be REM sleep, contradicting the conclusion of Salley (1982).

The level of physiological arousal seen during the out-of-body experience indicates a much lower level of arousal, one accompanied by muscular relaxation. Seventy-nine percent of our subjects considered themselves to be in a state of physical relaxation and mental calmness. Moreover, our study indicates that the majority of out-of-body experiences do not occur while dreaming; they ordinarily occur in a physically relaxed awake state, if anything, more similar to daydreaming or a hypnagogic state.

A typical REM dream will be more visual and vivid, less abstract, less like thinking, and from a psychoanalytic point of view, will contain mainly primary process mentation (Freud 1900). The out-of-body experience is essentially a secondary process experience, that is, much more like waking consciousness. In fact the clarity of the consciousness is commented on by most subjects in our study and by those in other studies (Green 1968). This state of consciousness is sometimes extraordinarily clear, with a vividness that is striking. For instance Fox (1962) states, "The vividness of life increased a hundredfold, never had the sea and sky and trees shown with such glamour and beauty, never had I felt so absolutely well, so clear-brained, so divinely powerful, so inexplicitly free!"

The REM dream has a changing and fragmented quality, usually without a rational, coherent, and logical flow of imagery and is often vague and confused. Recall is extremely difficult, and drop-off in recall after awakening is very rapid. In comparison the mode of thought in an out-of-body experience is quite logical (secondary process), and recall is generally not problematic.

Some of the more fantastic "astral projection" OBE states, in which there is a phantasmagoria of supersonic percepts, entities, and "Star Wars" scenarios (for example, Muldoon and Carrington 1977; Fox 1962) seem very similar to REM dream reports and may not be out-of-body experiences. In fact the statement, "My experience is more real than a dream," follows naturally from the fact that people are noting more secondary process than occurs in a typical night dream, where there is usually also an intense degree of involvement, so that the awareness of dreaming is usually absent. In the out-of-body experience, a sense of reality in relation to the physical body is always present, at least in our restricted definition of such a state (see Chapter One).

While it would be specious to attempt to make an exact distinction between the out-of-body and REM dream state, it appears that future research might attempt to define the continuum on which these two experiences occur. For example the psychophysiologist in the dream laboratory is very often more interested in physiology and far less interested in the psychology of dreaming. The psychodynamically oriented dream scholar often has little interest in physiology. Some common ground needs to be found before such questions can be answered. REM dream reports emerging from psychophysiology laboratories are notoriously sparse in content since almost never are associations to the dream content asked for by the physiologically oriented psychologists. For this reason it may be premature to compare and contrast REM dream reports collected in the laboratory with what has been called "astral projection."

Two final points of differentiation between the OBE and the REM dream deserve mention. First, it is far less common for individuals to see themselves in a REM dream than it is in an out-of-body experience. In a typical REM dream, the issue of being the dreamer never arises. The second differential point is that typically, the REM dream contains highly condensed and dramatized symbolic material, partially subject to secondary revision by the ego (Sharpe 1961), to make it more logical and easier to remember and to defend against conflictual material in the dream. The OBE experience is rarely conflictual so less disguise is needed. As fewer of the dream mechanisms are required, there is correspondingly less secondary revision.

Paul Federn's (1952) contributions to understanding the dynamics of sleep illuminate the complex relationship between "body" and "mind" that occurs in both the OBE and the REM dream. These matters will be discussed in considerable detail in Chapter Ten.

Table 6.4 compares the REM dream with the typical out-of-body experience.

THE LUCID DREAM

What is a lucid dream? The term has had a wide variety of diverse synonyms, including dreams of knowledge, visions with out-of-body experiences, and astral projection. Lucid dreams were named by Van Eeden, a Dutch physician, who began a study of his own dreams in 1896. He became interested in a certain kind of dream in which he was aware of dreaming while the dream continued, and he called it a lucid dream. He read a paper to the British Psychical Research Society on this subject in 1913. By then he had recorded 500 dreams, approximately 70 percent were lucid. Van Eeden highlighted certain features of lucid dreams; for example, a high positive association between lucid dreams and dreams of flying or floating in the air. The lucid dream was frequently followed by a nonlucid dream from which he would wake up. Waking from a lucid dream was rare unless it was preprogrammed (Van Eeden 1913).

The phenomenon of astral catalepsy (Fox 1962), that is, the "paralytic state of being aware while dreaming," which Fox and a number of others, including Muldoon, Carrington, and Monroe, feel is a necessary precondition for inducing out-of-body experiences, might actually be a lucid dream state. Very little reference to lucid dreaming can be found in the traditional literature. In our survey the term lucid dreaming was not referenced at all in such authoritative texts as *Kramer's Dream Psychology and the New Biology of Dreaming*, (1969), and *The Mind in Sleep* by Arkin et al. (1978). In contrast lucid dreaming has captured the imagination of the parapsychological and metaphysical community with best-selling publications on the control of dreaming, on learning to stop dreams, and on

Table 6.4
A COMPARISON OF REM DREAMS
AND OUT-OF-BODY EXPERIENCE

REM Dreams	OBEs
Occur when sleeping as part of a rhythmic sleep-dream 90-minute cycle.	Typically occur when awake. No known cycle.
Consciousness is often hazy and confused.	Consciousness is clear and often vivid.
Unreality of dream is accepted after awakening.	Reality of OBE is asserted emphatically.
Physical body not usually seen.	Physical body usually seen.
Little or no sense of being separate from the dream. Only experiencing self is active.	Usually observing and experiencing selves are integrated and active.
Regular tonic and phasic autonomic function with desynchronized EEG and Rapid Eye Movements.	No tonic-phasic variability. No rapid Eye Movement. EEG not desynchronized.
Sexual arousal usual.	Sexual arousal unusual.
Mainly primary process mentation.	Mainly secondary process mentation.
Recall difficult; secondary revision.	Recall easy; little secondary revision.
Only occasionally very pleasant; rarely life-changing.	Usually very pleasant; often life-changing.

dreaming the world in Carlos Castaneda's famous set of books about the training of an anthropologist from the United States in Yaqui Mexican Indian sorcery (1972). Faraday's books, *Dream Power* (1972) and *The Dream Game* (1974), have a less mystical flavor. Contrary to references in the literature (Sparrow 1975), lucidity in dreams is probably quite common, based on our informal surveys of students and on our clinical experience.

In a lucid dream there is little discontinuity with ordinary experience, a strong sense of integrated self, both observing and experiencing, and an intrinsic rationality within the dream, with a preservation of distance and objectivity. Complex cognitive activity is possible in the lucid dream state, especially with practice. Sparrow (1975), in his studies of his own lucid dreams, is able to enter meditative and prayer states without interrupting the process of the dreaming itself. Tasks irrelevant to the actual dream can be performed by practiced lucid dreamers. For example LaBerge (1980; LaBerge et al. 1981) was able to train five subjects to signal physically while they were lucid dreaming. One subject transmitted his initials in Morse code by tensing and relaxing his fists, demonstrating that complex motor and cognitive activity is possible.

The "lucidity" of the lucid dream and the "lucidity" of the out-of-body experience bear comparison. The clarity of consciousness is consistently reported by OBE experimenters (Green 1968a; Fox 1962; Whiteman 1956), who say the individual feels "alive at last after a physical life that in comparison seems like a dream or prison" (p. 274). Others, such as Muldoon and Carrington (1977, pp. 28-29), some of Monroe's (1977) accounts, and Crookall's (1965) cases, describe a transformative feeling in the lucidity of consciousness during the out-of-body state, as if the lucidity outstrips that of normal waking consciousness. Sparrow (1975) also states, "Once the lucidity has been initiated, either through emotional stress or the activation of the critical facility, the dreamer usually experiences a qualitative change in the dream. There is usually a tremendous sense of personal freedom and independence."

The sort of lucidity described by Sparrow, Fox, and others has mystical or noetic qualities that make this perception rather similar to the classical noetic mystical experiences described by William James (1961). Many people in our studies do not describe this mystical lucidity when they have OBEs. For example the research scientist described at the beginning of this chapter found the out-of-body state little different from that of being ordinarily awake. Others have described a certain amount of dreamlike confusion in the out-of-body state. There is considerable confusion in the theosophical literature generated by the "OBE as a lucid dream" argument because of the authoritative impact of the classical out-of-body "travelers" such as

Fox and Muldoon. Their concept is that astral catalepsy is a necessary precondition for the classic out-of-body effect. These are anecdotal opinions only, and, like so many opinions, have become reified by the authority of the individual. There is no scientific evidence to support such claims.

Some writers, such as Crookall (1965), feel that there is a "blanking out period" between being "in-the-body" and being "out-of-the-body," certainly far from a state of lucidity. Crookall's findings, while anecdotal, were based on systematic surveys of large numbers of subjects. One frequent feature of lucid dreams is captured in Freud's reported comments on Hervey de Saint-Denys, (LaBerge 1981), the famous lucid dreamer of the nineteenth century: "It seems as though in (the lucid dreamer's case) the wish to sleep has given way to another...wish, namely to observe his dreams and enjoy them." In fact lucid dreamers can program and, in experienced cases, produce their own dreams at will, somewhat like writing the script, directing, selecting the cast, and actually performing in a movie. LaBerge (1981) has called the lucid dream the "magic theater of all possibilities."

The lucid dreaming state is represented by the conclusion "I am dreaming," implying a realization that the dream is an outgrowth of one's own mental content. Thus, the dream is implicitly seen as being personal, a production of the individual's mind. The out-of-body experiencer, however, tends to endorse a more objective rather than a subjective view of reality, usually on the level of physical reality. The OBEer is very much in an observer role and implicitly has accepted a subject-object division: "I am here, and my body is down there." The person having an out-of-body experience is more likely to consider the phenomenal realm to be independent of the OBEer, just as material reality is, and the OBEer assumes a passive role in the experience in contrast to the lucid dreamer, whose role is both active and subjective. Unpleasant out-of-body experiences, for example, may be seen as objective and hence not within the experiencer's control. The out-of-body experience may lead to a naive and pathological avoidance of unpleasant experience. On the other hand, the naive lucid dreamer may also be trapped by denial of alien and negative psychopathological imagery.

In one survey of lucid dreams (Gackenbach 1979), 90 subjects were studied over a one-month period for personality attributes and cognitive style. The lucid dreams themselves were found to be structurally dissimilar to other dreams, especially in the degree of perceived control of the dreamer. Frequent lucid dreamers tended to score lower on measures of neuroticism and anxiety and also were more field independent.

In two studies by Blackmore (1982) of 217 students, 79 percent reported lucid dreams. All of these students had had at least one out-of-body experience. In a second study 14 percent of a sample of 115 students reported OBEs, and 73 percent reported lucid dreams. Only in the first of Blackmore's two studies were the out-of-body experiences and lucid dreams likely to be reported by the same people, and in neither study were out-of-body experiences or lucid dreams related to frequency of dream recall. Lucid dreams were frequently also flying dreams. Attempts were made by Blackmore to distinguish the lucid dreamers from out-of-body experiencers using two questionnaire instruments designed to assess mental imagery and its control. There was, however, no significant relationship between these scores and the reporting of either out-of-body experiences or lucid dreams. Other more randomly controlled surveys of the incidence of lucid dreaming, such as Palmer's (1979), found that 59 percent of the townspeople and 71 percent of the students claimed to have had lucid dreams, many of them regularly. Green (1966) found that 73 percent of a student sample had lucid dreams, while Kohr (1980) came up with a similar figure (70 percent).

Little electroencephalographic information is available on the lucid dream, though LaBerge et al. (1981) report a study of four subjects: "Lucid dreams occurred at times of unambiguous REM sleep. There was, however, occasional alpha rhythm and the possibility that the lucid dream is a variant of what could be called micro-awakenings remains, although lucid dreaming does occur without the presence of such alpha rhythms."

Celia Green (1968b) makes certain distinctions between the lucid dream and the out-of-body experience: 1) the out-of-body experience usually starts when the subject is awake rather than asleep, as compared with the lucid dream, which starts when the subject is already asleep; 2) the out-of-body experiencer considers what he or she is seeing as congruent with the real physical world, whereas the lucid dreamer regards the dream production as less identical with the physical world, that is, there is awareness that an "unreal" dream is occurring; 3) the lucid dream tends to contain more fantastic and symbolic elements than the OBE; 4) the visual field of the lucid dream tends to be blurred or indistinct as compared with the visual field of the out-of-body experience; 5) the extent to

Table 6.5
COMPARISON OF LUCID DREAMS AND OBE

Lucid Dream	OBE
50-70% incidence in general population.	14-25% incidence in general population.
Occurs only during sleep.	Occurs usually when awake.
Dreamer can consciously program the dream.	OBEer is a passive, objective observer.
Dreamer and his physical body are still integrated.	OBEer perceives himself as separated from his physical body, which is inert and thoughtless.
Consciousness often vivid, with mystical qualities in experienced subjects.	Consciousness more ordinary, like being awake, even in experienced subjects.
Dream is seen as a totally personal (subjective) production of the dreamer's mind.	OBEer does not see it as a subjective personal production, but rather as objective reality.
EEG; REM dream type with occasional alpha.	No typical REM findings on EEG.
Physical body not visible.	Physical body usually visible.
Fewer have a lasting positive impact.	Usually a highly positive lasting impact.

which the out-of-body experiencer can freely move through space and the intensity of the positive emotional state is generally greater than that of the lucid dreamer; and 6) in the out-of-body experience, individuals feel disembodied and believe that they occupy a position in space where they can act as observers of their physical bodies. This is uncommon in lucid dreams, where the physical body is very real, and the person is "inside" of it, often aware of bodily sensations and capable of making complex integrated bodily movements such as those reported by LaBerge et al. (1981). Table 6.5 summarizes the differences between the out-of-body state and the lucid dream.

DAYDREAMING

Popular misconceptions about psychiatric illness have often characterized patients, especially schizophrenic patients, as people lost in a world of fantasy. Studies of daydreaming in patients who have severe psychiatric illness (Starker and Singer 1975) show no relation whatsoever between daydream style and psychiatric symptoms. An out-of-body experience might be considered to be the product of fantasy even if the individual is not considered to be psychotic. It is sometimes felt that the OBE is being imagined in the way a daydream is imagined. Let us then consider the nature of daydreaming.

As William James (1950) said: "The first fact for us...is that thinking of some sort goes on...it seems as if the elementary psychic fact were not thought, or this thought or that thought but my thought, every thought being owned" (pp. 224-25). Daydreaming is a very personal form of imagery. An extensive and growing body of empirical research (Singer and Pope 1980) has made it increasingly clear that daydreaming and related forms of reverie are widespread, naturally occurring experiences in normal individuals (Singer 1966, 1975). Daydreaming in fact is a daily occurrence, with cultural variations in content or acceptance. Giambra (1982) examined 112 white and 112 black people. Significant differences were found between the two groups in achievement-oriented and hostile daydreams, differences thought to be due to the effect of the existence of a black minority culture within a white majority culture, whereas the basic elements of the OBE and NDE are consistent across cultures (Shiels 1978).

Klinger (1978) usefully defines a daydream as "spontaneous fantasy with a plot not based on current reality with qualities of being stimulus-independent," that is, not related to what is going on in the outside world but generated in the mind. Extensive studies using the retrospective questionnaire approach to daydreaming have differentiated three rather distinct types of daydreamers through factor analysis of randomly selected, large samples of normal daydreamers (Singer 1975): 1) the tortured, self-examining, driven-to-achievement and heroic accomplishment type, who have a generally negatively toned fantasy life; 2) anxious, self-doubting, fearful, disorganized individuals, who do not have clear and elaborate daydreams, and who may be oriented around possible failure (these two types seem similar to Shapiro's (1965) obsessional personality and anxious hysterical personality styles, respectively); 3) the third style that Singer has described represents a positive orientation toward internal experience, acceptance of it, and interest in one's own visual and orderly imagery capacities. It does not relate to any standard form of psychiatric illness. Daydreaming, as Giambra (1974) indicates, does vary over the life span. Daydreaming of the guilt-ridden, anxious variety generally declines with increasing age. No decline with age is noted for the more positive forms of daydreaming. In Giambra's studies future-oriented daydreaming does decline somewhat with age, as do sexual fantasies.

Grotstein (in press) notes that in psychotic and severe borderline patients, fantasy and daydreaming are inhibited. The patient is often overwhelmed by alien thoughts generated by psychotic processes, causing suppression of fantasy and daydreaming.

The type of thinking used by the average individual in the course of normal wakefulness can be quite variable. Attempts have been made to classify thinkers according to the styles they use. Ninety-five percent of people can form a visual image in full wakefulness when given a specific instruction (Horowitz 1970). Attempts have also been made to classify people according to verbal visual style (Richardson 1969). Out-of-body experiencers, at least in some studies, tend to be nonvisual in their styles (Irwin 1980), and certainly in the prototypical out-of-body experience, subjects emphasize position in space, sense of energy and movement, and a variety of overwhelmingly positive emotional states, rather than the visual phenomena.

As Horowitz (1970) indicates, mental images can increase when planfulness decreases and persons enter a state of directionless thought. Some people do so deliberately while meditating. In meditative states the flow of thoughts generally slows down and eventually ceases. This point at which the mind stops is considered in many systems to be the beginning of the meditative practice itself (Brown 1977) and is often associated with a variety of intense emotional, mystical, and nirvana states. It is not, however, associated with out-of-body experiences, which, if reported during meditation, are usually reported only in the very early phases, where the thinking is active, logical, and goal-directed (Twemlow, unpublished data).

There has been extensive work attempting to correlate certain behaviors with daydreaming scales. One such study (Antrobus et al. 1967) shows that frequent daydreamers also tend to be more distractable when they are performing a particular task and hence make more errors in such tasks. Similar work has indicated that there are types of people who are increasingly attentive to their inner, private processes and at times may prefer to live there than in the external world. The more the subject is absorbed in daydreaming, the less aware the subject is of the outside world. Isaacs (1975) shows that people who have high numbers of positive and vivid daydreams are also more likely to speak metaphorically and analogically when describing their daydreams.

The wish-fulfilling quality of daydreams is reported by Freud (1908). He clearly indicates that in the creative writer there is often a memory of an earlier experience that motivates creativity. Freud compared adult daydreaming with child's play, which he considered to be determined by wishes. Freud believed the dominant wish motivating play in children is the wish to grow up, while in the adult, it is the wish to be famous or successful. In general the motive force of fantasies is unsatisfied wishes, and every fantasy is the fulfillment of a wish, that is, a correction of an unsatisfying reality.

A variety of other studies have been made of daydreaming under special conditions. Prisoners, for example, have more sadistic and escape fantasies (Beit-Hallahmi 1972). Hariton and Singer (1974) showed that women who were brought up in more conventional and conservative ways were more likely to use daydreams of being raped in order to develop sexual arousal during intercourse with their husbands.

Daydreaming also serves a modestly arousing function. In experimental studies Antrobus (1968) found that daydreaming kept subjects awake by varying the content during long and monotonous tasks. Actually, much of the research on daydreaming demonstrates that daytime mentation is by no means organized and structured as most people have assumed. In Freud's sense secondary process thinking is not characteristic of all wakeful cognitive processes. Many researchers in mental imagery, for example, Singer (1975) and Antrobus (1968), take an information-processing approach to the problem of waking thought, including daydreaming. They consider, in William James' sense, that "stream of consciousness" is a more accurate depiction of the way normal waking thinking occurs. This concept of a stream of consciousness is used because it evokes images of thought flowing as a stream with a complex interplay between external input information and recalled information stored on a long-term basis in a reverberating circuit. Table 6.6 summarizes the main differences between an out-of-body experience and a daydream.

TWILIGHT STATES: HYPNAGOGIC AND HYPNOPOMPIC IMAGERY

The sort of imagery that occurs in that twilight area between being asleep and awake has been the subject of intensive study by a number of authors over several decades. Richardson (1969) feels that imagery experiences while falling asleep (hypnagogic imagery) and

Table 6.6
A COMPARISON OF THE DAYDREAM AND THE OBE

Daydreams	OBEs
Common if not daily occurrences.	Somewhat unusual occurences.
Occur in 100 percent of population.	Occur in 15–25 percent of population.
Manifestly wishfulfilling.	Not clearly wishfulfilling.
Often have ruminative quality.	No ruminative elements.
Highly subjective quality to the imagery.	Objective quality to imagery.
Known to be imagined by the daydreamer.	Reality of the OBE is emphasized.
Significantly culturally influenced.	Not significantly culturally affected.
Personality style influences imagery.	Personality style not correlated with the experience.
Declines with age.	Occurs at any age.
Frequent daydreamers tend to be visualizers.	OBEers not usually visualizers.
More like primary process thinking.	More like secondary process thinking.
Future oriented.	Usually present oriented.

upon waking (hypnopompic imagery), are phenomenologically similar to perceptual isolation imagery (Vernon 1963), hallucinogenic drug imagery (Thale 1950), photic stimulation imagery (Freedman 1965), sleep deprivation imagery (Bliss 1962), and meditation imagery (Pincard 1957). Hypnagogic images can occur in any sensory modality. The main defining characteristic is that they occur in the time between wakefulness and sleep. The term is attributed to Alfred Maury, a French dream investigator. He used the term "illusion hypnagogique" (1861). The term hypnopompic imagery was first used by Myers in 1903 to describe imagery occurring in the drowsy state between sleeping and awakening.

There are no striking differences between hypnagogic and hypnopompic imagery. Types of images that might occur are often patches of light, geometric forms, single objects without backgrounds, like faces, and occasionally integrated scenes like landscapes. Their major characteristics are that they tend to be autonomous, visual, and meaningful and that the images appear and follow their own course independent of the experiencer's will. As McKellar (1957) observes, "They might surprise their authors by their highly creative and unreproductive character." If visual, they are more often vividly colored and appear with marked distinctiveness of detail. They are of brief duration, ranging from a fraction of a second to a couple of minutes, and often succeed one another in rapid succession. Changes in shape and size are not uncommon. Often the imagined face or object may drift across the visual field or appear to approach closer and closer from some position directly in front of the observer. These movements are, in fact, often associated with movements of the eyes.

The reported prevalence of this imagery varies considerably from study to study. A large-scale, random sample of 600 normal volunteer subjects between the ages of 20 and 80 showed that both types of experiences, that is, hypnagogic and hypnopompic, were reported by a majority of subjects (Richard et al. 1981). Hypnagogic imagery was more common in women and subjects of lower social class. Hypnopompic imagery showed no such differences. Neither type of experience was associated with either verbal or nonverbal intelligence. Other estimates are not as high. Leaning (1926) estimates that about one-third of the general population have at some time had a visual hypnagogic image. A study by McKellar and Simpson in 1954 reported that 35 percent of Aberdeen University students had had vivid visual images in the half-awake state that precedes sleep. In McKellar's study auditory type hypnagogic images were slightly more frequent. The hypnagogic image, whether auditory, visual, or other sensory modality, is experienced as extremely real. It is probably this feature that most often leads to confusion with the out-of-body experience. The out-of-body experience appears not to be related to social class, and there is no clear skewing in sex distribution.

Personality attributes and psychophysiological measures of the hypnagogic and hypnopompic state have not been definitively demonstrated. However, Foulkes (1966) defines the hypnagogic state by an EEG measure. His subjects were "in descending stage 1 sleep, predominantly alpha." The most dreamlike hypnagogic imagery was found to be present in psychologically healthy people as measured by the California Personality Inventory and from the Thematic Apperception Test (TAT). These subjects had greater social poise, were less rigidly conformist, and were more self-accepting. They also showed greater creative achievement. Those who had low hypnagogic imagery had a typical authoritarian syndrome. They were more rigid, conventional, and intolerant. REM sleep state ratings were found to be uncorrelated with the ratings obtained during hypnagogic states. Foulkes' view of the hypnagogic image is characterized best in his own words, "an ego controlled excursion into inner thoughts and feelings, following the ego's voluntary decathexis of sensory input from the external world. Subjects with egos lacking adequate defenses against impulse life tend to be overwhelmed by it during REM sleep, hence experience especially vivid REM sleep dreams."

From a psychiatric point of view, it has often been said that hypnagogic states are more common in depressed (Starker et al. 1975) and hysterical people (Freedman et al. 1975). Hypnagogic and hypnopompic hallucinations are also part of the classical syndrome of narcolepsy, a condition characterized by excessive daytime sleepiness, brief unexpected sleep attacks, cataplexy, sleep paralysis, and hypnagogic and hypnopompic hallucinations (Zorick et al. 1979). Tricyclic antidepressants can also cause hypnagogic and hypnopompic hallucinations (Schlauch 1979).

Isakower (1938) described peculiar bodily distortions often involving the mouth as occasionally characteristic of the hypnagogic state in normal individuals and in certain borderline and psychotic states. The out-of-body phenomenon seems to show no particular dominance of visual or auditory imagery. In fact spatial sense and the sense of movement seem to be more striking modalities in the out-of-body state. As Foulkes says (1966), "In our experience, hypnagogic images are quite often believed to represent experiences actually taking place in the 'real world,' and they often involve the self in an active role." Very often in the hypnagogic state a single sensation, often a voice or a visual image, is real and the rest of the experience is dreamlike. This contrasts with the out-of-body experience, where the whole experience is real. Hypnagogic and hypnopompic hallucinations are also associated with paresthesias in the mouth and hands (Freedman et al. 1975) and vague visual images often of large objects approaching and receding. These are not phenomena characteristic of the out-of-body experience.

A 59-year-old white woman who was being treated with amitryptiline for depression and propranolol for mild chronic heart disease, can clearly differentiate dreaming from lucid dreaming and from hypnagogic and hypnopompic imagery. She says that in the lucid dream the transition between dreaming and being aware of dreaming is sudden as compared with the confused state often present in hypnopompic imagery. She is certain that during her hypnopompic states her eyes are open. The process of seeing is different. She says, "Dreaming is in the mind." This report is in stark contrast with the sense of objectivity in the out-of-body experience.

Sometimes increased hypnagogic phenomena are present as a prelude to a psychotic episode. A 45-year-old paranoid schizophrenic professional man reports that prior to a psychotic episode he experiences the following, "Before I am going to have trouble, just as I drop off to sleep...I wouldn't exactly call them hallucinations, though they are visual, I see letters and numbers, for example, X612, then I know that I am going to have trouble with my thinking that night." This report is an example of the clearly defined feature of autonomy with hypnagogic imagery (Gordon 1949, 1962), meaning that the imagery comes of its own accord and can be surprising in content. In this sense it is similar to dreams and hallucinations and quite different from the out-of-body experience, which is usually a controlled phenomenon.

McKellar (1972) notes that in both hypnagogic and hypnopompic states, body image disturbances can occur. Often, part or all of a person's body has grown or shrunk in size or has become in some way distorted, and these distortions often give rise to anxiety and terror. Such experiences of distortion of body imagery are quite uncommon in the out-of-body experience. In addition the hypnopompic state, which is slightly less common than the hypnagogic state because of its association with sleep, is often characterized by strange subvocalizations called by McKellar "hypnopompic speech," thought by many to represent a commentary on dream imagery. McKellar quotes the example of a young woman who to her surprise awoke murmuring "put the pink pajamas in the salad." Such nonsensical speaking is not present in the out-of-body experience.

Occasionally, hypnagogic and hypnopompic imagery is called "hallucinatory." While many clinicians prefer to confine the term hallucination to disease states, authoritative sources such as Freedman et al. (1975) consider that, "A dream is a simple example of an hallucination." Hallucination is defined as "...the apparent perception of an external object when no corresponding real object exists—that is, an internal psychological event is mistakenly attributed to an external source" (p. 807).

Table 6.7
COMPARISON OF HYPNAGOGIC AND HYPNOPOMPIC IMAGERY WITH OBE

Hypnagogic and Hypnopompic Imagery	OBE
Usually visual or auditory with fragmented images occurring in rapid succession.	Usually spatial with integrated imagery.
Changes in shape and size of image is common.	Imagery unvaried.
Body image disturbances common.	Body image disturbances unusual.
Experienced commonly by general population.	Experienced less commonly by population.
More common in women (hypnagogic).	Even sex distribution.
More common in hysteria and depression.	No evidence of association with psychopathology.
Dreamlike and hazy except for the dominant image.	Whole experience clear and vivid.

Carr (1982), writing on near-death experiences, differentiates real and pseudohallucinations on the basis that in the former there is objectivity, while in the latter there is subjectivity. Thus, in Carr's opinion, the real and vivid quality of the NDE does not establish its reality, but more likely that it is simply a real hallucination. In the depths of psychosis, the hallucination *is* happening and, on these grounds alone, the reality of the OBE and NDE is hard to distinguish—both are vivid, compelling and intense. However, the psychotic who is that disturbed has other features of psychosis such as thought disorder, anxiety, etc. not present in OBE or NDE subjects, who usually function in a more integrated way (Greyson 1983). Table 6.7 distinguishes hypnagogic and hypnopompic states from the out-of-body experience.

CONCLUSION

In this chapter and the three preceding it, we have attempted to distinguish the out-of-body experience from pathological syndromes and from other states of consciousness. We are aware that these states cannot be absolutely distinguished, and more likely represent a continuum on a spectrum of consciousness, as we will propose in some detail in Chapter 10. At the same time, for reasons of accurate differential diagnosis and treatment planning, we feel it is important to delineate these preliminary distinctions, from both a descriptive and a clinical point of view. In Chapters 3, 4, and 5, where the OBE is distinguished from depersonalization, autoscopy and schizophrenic boundary loss, we make no claim that people who experience these psychopathological states can not have out-of-body experiences as well. They can. The important point here is that such phenomena are not synonymous with depersonalization, autoscopy, or psychosis, nor are they the same as dreams, twilight states, or daydreams.

Part III
THE NEAR-DEATH EXPERIENCE

Seven — AN OVERVIEW OF THE NEAR-DEATH EXPERIENCE

No instance of altered mind/body perception has attracted as much popular attention as the near-death experience. This chapter is the first of three that explore this special and dramatic example of the out-of-body experience. Since the publication of Raymond Moody's *Life After Life* (1975), the media has seized upon the near-death experience (NDE) and exploited it to the hilt. Movies and television specials have been made on the subject, and paperback books filled with anecdotal accounts have rushed into print. The experience is familiar by now and is summarized in composite form by Moody:

> A man is dying and, as he reaches the point of greatest physical distress, he hears himself pronounced dead by the doctor. He begins to hear an uncomfortable noise, a loud ringing or buzzing, and at the same time feels himself moving very rapidly outside his own physical body, but still in the same immediate physical environment, and sees his own body from a distance as though he is a spectator. He watches the resuscitation attempts from this vantage point and is in a state of emotional upheavel.
>
> After a while, he collects himself and becomes more accustomed to his odd condition. He notices that he still has a 'body,' but one of a very different nature and with very different powers from the physical body he has left behind. Some other things begin to happen. Others come to meet him and help him. He glimpses the spirits of relatives and

friends who have already died, and the loving, warm spirit of a kind he has never encountered before—a being of light—appears before him. This being asks him a question, nonverbally, to make him evaluate his life and helps him along by showing him a panoramic, instantaneous playback of the major events of his life. At some point, he finds himself approaching some sort of barrier or border, apparently representing the limit between earthly life and the next life. Yet, he finds that he must go back to earth, that the time for his death has not yet come. At this point he resists, for by now he is taken up with his experiences in the afterlife and does not want to return. He is overwhelmed by intense feelings of joy, love, and peace. Despite his attitude, though, he is somehow united with his physical body and lives (1975, pp. 23-24).

REVIEW OF THE SCIENTIFIC LITERATURE

In recent years these experiences have begun to come under the scrutiny of systematic scientific investigation, and in addition to the anecdotal reports of Moody and others, we now have a number of reports in the literature derived from methodologies that are more or less scientific (Noyes 1972; Noyes and Kletti 1976a; Noyes and Kletti 1976b; Noyes and Kletti 1977a; Noyes and Kletti 1977b; Ring 1980; Sabom 1982; Gabbard, Twemlow, and Jones 1981; Twemlow, Gabbard, and Coyne 1982; Greyson and Stevenson 1980). Of course not everyone who has a brush with death has a classical NDE or even a partial experience, characterized by only a few of the major components. Ring (1980) found that approximately 51 percent of illness and accident victims have an NDE, a figure not too divergent from that reported by Sabom and Kreutziger (1977), who found that 61 percent of 100 persons who had been unconscious while close to death had an NDE. Ring conceptualizes the near-death experience as unfolding in a five-stage continuum. The first stage involves a feeling of extraordinary peace and contentment; the second stage is characterized by a sense of detachment from one's physical body, that is, an OBE; the third stage is decribed as entering the transitional world of darkness; the hallmark of the fourth stage is a brilliant light of exceptional beauty; and the last stage is one in which the subject experiences himself or herself as "entering the light" (1980).

Although more than 60 percent of NDE subjects experience stage one, a steadily decreasing number of subjects experience each of the subsequent stages, tapering down to roughly 10 percent who describe stage five. Hence, in Ring's study the experience of being "out-of-body" was not necessarily a cardinal feature of the experience.

Greyson and Stevenson (1980) had somewhat different findings in their retrospective analysis of 78 cases of near-death experience. The impression of being outside of one's physical body was reported by 70 percent of their respondents. Of those subjects who reported out-of-body experiences as part of the NDE, 71 percent claimed they could see and hear persons physically present. Ninety-five percent reported that they seemed to be able to move about in the out-of-body state, and 77 percent had the impression of some sort of nonphysical body separate from the physical body. Thirty-one percent of their respondents had the impression of passing through a tunnel during the NDE, while 72 percent seemed to enter some unearthly realm of existence. A border or "point of no return," as described in Moody's book (1975) was reported by 57 percent of their subjects. Forty-nine percent reported that they met a person who was not physically present—27 percent identified this person as a "being of light" while 25 percent identified it as a religious figure, 16 percent a deceased acquaintance, 14 percent a living acquaintance, and 26 percent could not identify the individual. The so-called "panoramic memory" was reported by 27 percent of their subjects.

One of the most significant findings of the Greyson and Stevenson survey is the profound attitudinal changes accompanying an NDE. Seventy-five percent of their subjects reported significant changes in attitudes towards God or religion, 74 percent toward the self, 73 percent toward one's own death, and 72 percent toward death in general. Sixty-four percent had significant attitudinal changes about the meaning of life as a result of the NDE. These findings are consistent with those of Ring (1980) and the anecdotal reports of Moody (1975).

If there were any doubts about the pervasiveness of the near-death experience in the U.S. population, George Gallup, Jr., of Gallup Poll fame, has laid them to rest. Legitimate questions could be raised about the skewed nature of the samples of other NDE researchers. Those subjects who respond to advertising are a self-selected group, not typical of the population as a whole, one can argue. However, in his recent book, *Adventures in Immortality* (1982),

Gallup has utilized his considerable expertise in polling methods to survey 1,500 adult Americans, typical of the population at large. Although his term "verge of death experience" is not as precisely defined as most NDE researchers would like, his statistical findings are nonetheless quite impressive. Fifteen percent of the U.S. adult population have been close to death; and of this figure, equal to about 23,000,000 persons in the U.S. population, 35 percent report classical near-death experiences. In other words roughly 5 percent of the population of the United States has had an NDE. The same elements of the NDE described previously are present in his data. However, some of the percentages are lower than other studies would indicate. For example the out-of-body experience component was only present in 26 percent of those reporting near-death experience. These discrepancies may well be due to Gallup's broader and less precise definition. As in other studies, Gallup finds no relationship between the preexisting religious beliefs of the subject and the presence or form of the NDE. Demographic variables are not relevant to NDE subjects, according to Gallup, who found that these experiences occur in roughly equal distribution across categories of sex, race, education, area of the country, age, and income. Gallup's book is primarily a popular book aimed at delineating beliefs about immortality in the population. His chief relevance to NDE research, as Ring (1982) has pointed out, is that it has legitimized the NDE as a pervasive and consistent phenomenon through scientifically sound statistical methods.

CASE EXAMPLE

The figures from empirical studies fail to capture the dramatic, life-transforming quality of the individual experience. The preceding quotation from Moody is a composite experience, combining many different features from different individual reports. Rarely does one experience encompass all of those characteristics. The following example of a brush with death, experienced by a 24-year-old woman we shall call Miss N., is both representative of a typical NDE as well as unique in its individual idiosyncratic qualities. We report it in her own words so as to preserve the immediacy and subjectivity of the experience:

I had taken drugs on top of alcohol without knowing what I

was doing. I was taken to intensive care, where after a few days I felt I was rapidly going downhill and knew I would die. I began to pray that I would not die and felt myself losing consciousness. The doctors and nurses later told me that they lost my heartbeat for seven minutes. As I began to lose consciousness, I saw my life flash in front of me like an old movie with incredibly speeded-up action.

As soon as I died, I still had a mind as a matter of speaking. I did not have a physical body. It was more or less a soul or spirit. The first thing that happened was that I felt I was being lifted into the air. I was being transported through a strange atmosphere when all of a sudden I remember hearing the most beautiful heavenly music that I have ever heard. There was a rolling harp, a flute, and a xylophone. Then I was standing in front of a long, dark tunnel and began to worry how I would find my way out of it. Above and ahead of me, I noticed some light and an opening. I thought of going toward it, but very soon I noticed the opening coming closer and getting larger.

I looked again and felt my name being called out. There was a spirit form standing in the opening. To me it was some kind of angel or perhaps God. There was a white transparent type of robe or garb with a radiant gold belt around his waist. Where the face, hands and feet would normally appear, was a radiant light shining and glowing. This being gave me a very comforting feeling, and it did not exactly speak to me out loud. It was as though he was transmitting a message into my brain very clearly. He said I was too young and that it was not time for me to go. He said I had much to live for. I was to tell the people of the world that there is life after death and that there are higher beings and a God so they could be comforted by this information.

I came back to life after this being spoke with me and found myself in my body. At first, I did not realize I was in the hospital. The nurses told me I kept repeating over and over again, 'It's so beautiful.' I have never been the same since. I will never again fear death, and I now have a purpose and meaning to my life that I never had before.

This poignant experience not only catalogues the key phenomenological features of the NDE in this account, but also conveys a sense of the profound impact these experiences typically have on the life of the subject. A sense that a miracle has occurred is common, as is a conviction that the out-of-body experience is positive proof of the separation of the soul from the physical body. These convictions often lead to religious conclusions involving the existence of God, proof of life after death, and an increased religiosity in the subjects themselves. How can we account for the consistency of these elements across several different studies and even across cultures? Numerous hypotheses have been advanced.

EXPLANATORY HYPOTHESES

In approaching a systematic analysis of the explanatory hypotheses proposed for near-death experiences, one might first ponder the following question: Exactly what is it about the experience that must be explained? Grosso (1981) has suggested that three components of the near-death experience demand explanation: 1) the consistency and universality of the experience across cultures and across individuals; 2) the paranormal aspects of near-death experiences; and 3) the tendency for the NDE to transform values and attitudes. The various models put forth to explain the experience generally touch on one or more of these components, but no model provides a comprehensive and convincing explanation of all aspects of the near-death experience. In considering these hypotheses, it is important to keep in mind that they are only hypotheses. No definitive proof of causative factors in NDEs is yet available.

The explanatory models can be grouped into five general catagories: 1) cultural or religious programming; 2) birth models; 3) neurophysiological models; 4) psychological models; and 5) paranormal models. We shall consider each of these general models and critically examine their strengths and weaknesses.

Cultural or religious programming

When anecdotal accounts of NDEs first reached the public, it was widely suggested that such experiences are strongly programmed by the religious training and beliefs of the subject. Ever since childhood, when one learns in Sunday school that one's soul travels out of one's body to meet one's Maker following death, one gradually develops a mental set regarding what one can expect at the moment of death.

From this point of view, one might expect that NDEs are particularly prone to occur in individuals with strong religious inclinations. As one approaches the crisis of death, one might argue, the powerful wish-fulfilling fantasy stemming from one's religious background comes true in the vivid imagery of the NDE. However, the work of Osis and Haraldsson (1977), of Ring (1980), and of Gallup (1982) do not support this point of view. All studies indicate that preexisting religious beliefs do not affect the actual phenomenological content of the experience. The interpretation of the being of light seen in the near-death experience is influenced by one's religious background as seen in our preceding example. However, the actual phenomonological form of the experience is basically the same regardless of one's religious affiliation or beliefs. More about the interpretation of the symbols in the NDE will be discussed in Chapter Nine.

Even the refutation of this hypothesis by the empirical findings of scientific studies does not entirely dismiss the central thesis of this explanatory model. One might argue that the notion of life after death is so culturally pervasive that we all have the concept culturally programmed into our unconscious regardless of religious teachings. We live in a culture where the media bombards us with culturally held beliefs about the survival of physical death. Particularly in the last decade, reports in the media are so frequent that an "NDE consciousness" has been created in the public. With this popular mind set, one might argue, the person who has an NDE is simply living out the "script" that has been written for him or her by the media. As a rebuttal to this argument, NDEs have been shown to present a remarkable invariance across a variety of cultural, demographic, and personal parameters (Ring 1980; Gallup 1982). Perhaps an even more compelling rebuttal is contained in an examination of NDE reports from small children, which we will explore in some depth in Chapter Nine.

Birth Models

Of all the explanatory models for the near-death experience, one of the most popularized is the birth model, made famous by astronomer Carl Sagan, well-known popularizer of science, in his best selling book, *Broca's Brain* (1979). Borrowing from the work of Stanislav Grof (1975), who noted that the brilliant light typical of near-death experience is also found in mystical states and LSD trips, Sagan reduces the complexities of the near-death experience to a simple recapitulation of the birth experience. The primal memory of birth is shared by all human beings and therefore could explain the universality of the NDE in Sagan's view. The sensation of flight from the body is the ejection from the womb; the tunnel effect is a repetition of the infant's passage through the vaginal canal; the emergence from darkness into a brilliant light is, of course, the light of the delivery room; and the heroic figure connected with the light is simply the obstetrician delivering the baby. Sagan asserts that birth is the only common experience comprising all of these features, and in so doing he believes he has glibly solved the mystery of the NDE.

Becker (1982) has elegantly refuted the premises of Sagan's argument. Becker points out that newborn infants simply lack the capacity to distinguish visual percepts clearly enough to store any visual memory of the birth experience. Moreover, they have no conceptual framework on which to organize visual images. Becker also draws our attention to obvious dissimilarities between the birth experience and the NDE, for example, passage through the vaginal canal would hardly be tunnel-like from the newborn's point of view, the heroic "figure of light" would be experienced as a terrifying torturer rather than a loving, Godlike figure to the infant in the throes of the anxiety that accompany being jerked from the womb, and the presence of deceased friends and relatives in the NDE is not explained by the birth model, where these figures are absent. Moreover, Grosso (1981) notes that if Sagan is right in viewing the NDE as a recapitulation of the birth experience, then those persons who have difficult births should have frightening and difficult NDEs, not to mention those who had delivery by Caesarian Section. He makes the obvious point that while being born into the world is painful, leaving the world seems to be pleasant. These experiences are actually opposites rather than analogues.

Neurophysiological Models

Unless resuscitative measures are applied rapidly, a person undergoing cardiac arrest will soon develop cerebral anoxia. McHarg (1978) and Rodin (1980) both consider this compromised oxygen supply to the brain to be the primary determinant of the imagery of the near-death experience. Carr (1982) observes that NDEs strongly resemble complex hallucinations associated with limbic lobe dysfunction. He speculates that behaviorally active peptides, that is, endorphins, undergo alternations in the limbic lobe neurons and produce endogenous hallucinogens, which are responsible for the NDE. Siegel (1980) further advances this notion that a compromised central nervous system is the primary etiologic factor in the production of the near-death experience. He notes the similarities between NDE and drug-induced hallucinations, and he attributes the imagery of tunnels, bright lights, and so on to phosphenes, visual sensations arising from the discharge of neurons and eye structures.

The status of these neurophysiological models as explanatory of the NDE phenomenon is highly questionable. One would be hard pressed to question that the perception of the NDE imagery must be mediated through central nervous system structures and neurophysiological processes. All mental functioning is. As explanatory models designed to understand the causation of the NDE, however, these hypotheses are sorely reductionistic. First of all, Siegel makes a fundamental error in assuming that because certain perceived phenomena are similar, they can be presumed to have the same underlying cause. Phenomenological similarities abound in nature, without adherence to unicausality. There is also no compelling evidence that indicates that a person experiencing an NDE has a neural status that is similar to a person experiencing hallucinations induced by drugs. The anoxia theory becomes untenable when one reads of documented cases of NDEs in subjects who were fully oxygenated during the entire NDE (Ring 1980). Finally, these models fail to account for the reports by Sabom (1982) of accurate observations of resuscitation efforts by NDE subjects (although the nature of Sabom's evidence can be seriously criticized).

Psychological Models

Noyes and Kletti (1976a) invoke the psychological defense mechanism of depersonalization as the explanation for the near-death experience. With the imminent threat of physical destruction facing the organism, they propose, a defensive split occurs between an observing self and a functioning self. The observing self can watch what is happening at a "safe" distance and deny that the functioning self facing the threat is actually part of him or her. They suggest that there is inherent survival value in the Darwinian sense in this defensive maneuver, and that a calm, detached frame of mind is created from which to plan strategies of survival, such as turning the wheel in an imminent auto accident or grabbing for a limb if one is falling from a mountain.

Their formulation, however, is not a comprehensive explanatory hypothesis for near-death experiences. As defined and described in Chapter Three, the phenomenon of depersonalization is different from the out-of-body experience. The near-death experience as described by Moody (1975) is more likely a variant of the out-of-body experience rather than a variant of depersonalization. While it is true that an accident victim may defensively split into an observing self and a functioning self as he or she enters the accident, the Moody-type NDE involves subjects who lose consciousness following the impact and find themselves floating above their limp bodies. In this regard we might well speak of a "before-death" experience, which Noyes and Kletti are referring to when they speak of depersonalization and an "after-death" experience, which is the Moody-type NDE described by most NDE researchers, that is, an out-of-body experience following loss of consciousness.

In their study of 189 survivors of life-threatening danger, they studied the responses through factor analysis. Noyes (1981) reports three emerging factors as a result of this analysis. Factor 1 was a mystical factor, factor 2 was a depersonalization factor, and factor 3 was a hyperalertness factor. Hyperalertness items were reported most frequently (59 percent), followed by depersonalization items (mean 39 percent), and mystical items were reported least frequently (26 percent). Noyes comments that the hyperalertness dimension is essentially the opposite of depersonalization, that is, hyperalertness factors are manifestations of heightened arousal in the face of a threatening environment while depersonalization is a dissociation of consciousness from that arousal. Together, they may represent an adaptive mechanism that combines opposing reaction tendencies, the one serving to intensify alertness, and the other to dampen potentially disorganizing emotion. Certain of Noyes' subjects went beyond the depersonalization and hyperalertness phase, or the "before-death" experience and passed into the mystical dimension, or the "after-death" experience (Moody-type NDE). Noyes (1981) notes that this dimension seemed to involve a more extensive alteration in consciousness and exclusion of the surrounding environment from awareness. Intense visual imagery was characteristic of this dimension, as was essential harmony or unity and detachment from the body. Hence, even in this population there is clear indication of the Moody-type NDE in a portion of the population, although the explanatory formulation involving depersonalization is relatively limited to the early stages of the experience.

Other psychological explanations for the NDE include that of Ehrenwald (1978) who views the out-of-body experience occurring in the context of the NDE as a defense against the threat of death. He sees the threat to the organism as activating omnipotent fantasies of survival of death in a manner akin to hallucinatory wish fulfillment. Ehrenwald claims that all out-of-body experiences have one thing in common—a characteristic array of defenses designed to ward off anxiety originating from the threatened disintegration of the ego, from the breakdown of the body image, and from the fear of death.

Greyson (1981a, 1983) argues that Grosso's three components requiring explanation (1981) can all be explained using a psychological model. The conceptualization of the near-death experience as a type of regression in the service of the ego has a good deal of heuristic value in his view. The feeling of cosmic unity may recapitulate the loss of ego boundaries typical of the autistic and symbiotic stages of infantile development; the mystical ineffability may be connected with regression to a preverbal developmental period; and the profound personality change following the experience, he suggests, may come from the increased lability or impressionability of infancy (1983). He explains the out-of-body sensation as an extension of the defensive detachment seen in depersonalization, where one wants to disavow any connection with the endangered body. He also believes that the impression of being out of one's body may be a secondary revision of the actual experience, wherein subjects defensively reconstruct their experiences in a way that is less threatening than the total loss of control and helplessness that they actually felt. The life review is understood by Greyson as a reflection of anticipatory grieving over the impending loss of life. He likens it to the reminiscences of the elderly as they approach death.

Greyson believes that even the paranormal material sometimes connected with near-death experience provides further evidence for the notion that there is a psychological need-subserving aspect of the NDE. He points out that most cases of paranormal perception that appear authenic are related to the satisfaction of psychological needs. He thus makes a case that if paranormal perceptions or experiences can be documented in NDEs, this evidence would attest to the NDE function of satisfying psychological needs of the individual.

Whether or not the psychodynamic interpretation is fully explanatory of the near-death experience, the psychological meaning of the experience has tremendous significance for the integration of the NDE into the individual's life subsequent to the experience. Greyson points out that the positive personality changes ensuing from NDEs promote a reverence and appreciation for life that decreases suicidal thoughts (1981b). The fact that the euphoria and mystical peacefulness attained by so many subjects during a near-death experience do not lead to repeated attempts at suicide in an effort to return to the transcendental bliss of the NDE presents an intriguing paradox, which deserves further psychological investigation.

Greyson is modest in his appraisal of the usefulness of psychodynamic models. He makes no effort to "explain it away" in a reductionistic manner. He allows for the fact that other levels of interpretation, such as the neurophysiological, are valid and do not conflict with models proposed at the level of psychological meaning. He even suggests that his psychodynamic hypotheses are compatible with the notion that the NDE might be an encounter with an alternate reality.

Grosso (1981) is similarly concerned about "reductionistic" explanations of near-death phenomena. He proposes a Jungian hypothesis involving an "archetype of death," which he defines as "a collective psychic structure whose function is to assist a human personality during a major crisis of individuation" (Grosso 1981, pp. 54-55). He acknowledges that it would be premature to invoke the Jungian hypothesis as fully explanatory of near-death experience. However, he rather oddly asserts that this hypothesis is "nonreductionistic." Here it seems that Grosso reveals a misunderstanding of the concept of reductionism, which actually refers to the reducing of data to seeming equivalents that are less complex or developed. His own explanation is barely one step beyond a tautological statement. He relabels the experience as an "archetype of death," which amounts to reducing an extremely complex phenomena to a simpler concept, which is similarly lacking in explanatory power. Moreover, the acceptance of this model requires the acceptance of a number of Jungian concepts, which are highly controversial, including the notion of the archetype, the collective unconscious, and the idea that this archetype is instructive to the individual in paving the way toward a "healthy death."

Paranormal Models

Most of the explanatory hypotheses provided for the near-death experience assume that the experience is something other than the near-death experience survivor thinks it is. The typical survivor believes in the "reality" of the experience, that is, a soul or spirit has separated from the physical body, traveled outside of it, and returned. Many survivors are convinced of the survival of death following the NDE. Osis and Haraldsson (1977) are open to this possibility and assert that their data on deathbed visions across individuals and cultures is compatible with the survival hypothesis.

Since the NDE survivor was not truly dead, but only near death, it is doubtful that the study of near-death experiences will ever provide definitive data on the survival hypothesis. However, some data are accumulating on the critical issue of whether or not the "out-of-body" position during an NDE is truly an extracorporeal point of perception. Sabom (1982) studied 116 near-death survivors and focused his research largely on the hypothesis that the subjects report observations from an "out-of-body" position that is potentially verifiable. In his group of 116 subjects, 32 reported that they could observe events during their own resuscitations. While 26 of the 32 cases reported general, nonspecific observations, which were possibly compatible with the known facts in each case, 6 of the 32 were of a more detailed nature and permitted an in-depth comparison of the observed events with the actual resuscitative procedures. The latter were constructed from the medical records and then compared with the subjective reports. In these 6 cases the "out-of-body" observations matched with the actual events. In each of these cases Sabom ruled out the possibility that the description was based on prior general knowledge of cardiopulmonary resuscitative procedures, that it was a result of information subsequently passed on to the resuscitated patient, and that it could possibly be an actual physical observation made during the resuscitation effort. Sabom concludes that at least some persons who report near-death experience may be experiencing a form of "extrapsychic" perception that allows them to perceive accurately events in the physical environment with some kind of extrasensory or "extrabodily" mechanism. He rejects the notion, however, that this constitutes any evidence for or against the existence of an afterlife since these patients are never truly dead. These data are difficult to evaluate. We will return to these data in Chapter Thirteen.

In this review of the various explanatory hypotheses of near-death experiences, we have not attempted a thorough critical examination of each proposed thesis. In the last section of this book, we present a comprehensive conceptual framework with which to understand the OBE. A number of the considerations raised here about NDEs will be addressed directly or indirectly in that section. We share

Greyson's view (1981a) that the available data do not support a coherent unicausal explanation of the phenomenon. We suggest that a multicausal view is probably most productive in explaining each of the various elements of the experience (Gabbard and Twemlow 1981), as we will elaborate in Chapter Eleven.

OBE VERSUS NDE

From the vantage point of our interest in out-of-body experiences in the general sense, we became curious as to whether there were substantive differences between NDEs and typical OBEs. For example are there certain features of NDEs that are exclusive to such experiences? Are there discriminating characteristics that allow one to differentiate OBEs from NDEs? Or, alternatively, are out-of-body experiences that occur in nonlife-threatening situations essentially the same as those that occur near death? To answer these questions we analyzed our data, collected as described in Chapter One, in such a way as to shed some light on these questions. First of all, one of the most significant findings of our study was that the vast majority of OBEs, 90 percent in our sample, do not occur during an NDE. Only 10 percent (34) of our 339 subjects reporting OBEs described them as occurring in near-death states.

Univariate independent group t-tests were performed on our data to determine if there were any characteristics that were significantly more often associated with the near-death subjects as compared to the 90 percent of the sample who were not near death at the time of their OBE. The results indicate that although no characteristic of the OBE is exclusive to the NDE, certain features are impressive inasmuch as they are significantly more often associated with NDEs than with other OBEs (see Table 7.1).

A person undergoing an NDE is more likely to hear noises during the early stages of the experience ($dF=188$, $p<.001$) and more likely to feel that he or she is traveling through a tunnel ($dF=318$, $p<.0007$). These persons are also more apt to sense that there are other beings in nonphysical form with them ($dF=322$, $p<.0002$), particularly deceased people with whom they had a close emotional bond ($dF=28$, $p<.006$). Encounters with the communicative being described as a "brilliant light" and for whom there is a strong attraction are also significantly more likely to occur with a person who has an OBE near death ($dF=314$, $p<.0001$). Finally, there are statistically significant

Table 7.1
INDEPENDENT VARIABLE:
AT TIME OF OBE WERE YOU NEAR DEATH?

Dependent Variable	X	S.D.	t	dF	P
Noises during early stages of OBE					
Yes	1.222	.428	-4.051	188.0	.001
No	1.686	.465			
Traveling through a tunnel					
Yes	1.500	.508	-3.438	318.0	.0007
No	1.769	.422			
Aware of other beings in nonphysical form					
Yes	1.353	.485	-3.736	322.0	.0002
No	1.672	.470			
Were beings people close to you who had already died					
Yes	1.538	.508	-2.952*	28.1	.006
No	1.841	.366			
See brilliant light					
Yes	1.344	.482	-4.839	314.0	.0001
No	1.743	.438			
Purpose connected to experience					
Yes	1.125	.336	-4.211*	48.5	.0001
No	1.405	.491			
Life changed by experience					
Yes	1.206	.410	-2.564	309.0	.01
No	1.433	.496			
Spiritual or religious experience					
Yes	1.176	.387	-4.372*	47.5	.0001
No	1.495	.501			
Experience of lasting benefit					
Yes	1.064	.250	-3.287*	52.3	.002
No	1.234	.424			

* Heterogeneous variance.

1 = Yes, 2 = No.

differences in the aftereffects of the experience if it occurs near death. The person is more likely to feel that there is a purpose connected to the experience (dF=48, p<.0001), that it is an experience of lasting benefit (dF=52, p<.002), that it is a spiritual or religious experience (dF=47, p<.0001), and that his or her life is changed by the experience (dF=309, p<.01).

These distinguishing features of the near-death experience are remarkably similar to those reported in Moody's anecdotal accounts (1975), Ring's survey (1980), and the study of Greyson and Stevenson (1980). Notably absent from the list are the experiences of peace and serenity, which are just as common in OBE as in NDE. Also absent are the experience of the panoramic life review and the experience of encountering a border or barrier beyond which the subject could not go. The absence of these elements could be related to the fact that the total N for each variable ranged from 326 through 30, and the reliability of differences, of course, varies proportionately. Interestingly, there was also no difference on the variable that measured change in belief about life after death. Sixty-six percent of all OBE subjects became more convinced that there was life after death, regardless of the proximity to death, indicating that the perception of the existence of consciousness as separate from the body may be the key factor influencing belief change, rather than any specific NDE characteristics.

No NDE feature was exclusive to the OBE that occurs near death. Each discriminating characteristic was also found in small numbers in subjects with OBEs originating in other preconditions. Hence, one cannot conclude from our results that NDEs are characterized by exclusive features that are not present in other forms of OBE. However, one can conclude that there are a number of distinguishing features that may differentiate NDEs from other OBEs in a statistically significant manner. Our data certainly support the idea that the NDE is special and unique when compared with other experiences where one perceives one's mind as separated from one's body.

Our data correlate well with other studies on NDE. The repeated emergence of these common denominators of the NDE lends further credence to the notion that the experience is one with a certain degree of universality and a characteristic array of elements associated with it. The results of our study suggest that the NDE cannot be written off as simply a typical OBE, bearing no relationship to survival threat. The proximity to death seems to provide it with certain characteristic features that differentiate it from other similar experiences.

Eight — THE CONTEXT OF THE NEAR-DEATH EXPERIENCE

In Chapter Seven we gave detailed consideration to the phenomenology of the near-death experience. Now we will consider the question of whether or not the NDE shows any variation in the descriptive features depending on the conditions that existed at the time of the experience. Although much research has impressionistically documented that the experience is fairly invariant across cultures (Becker 1981) and across religions (Lundahl 1983), a number of people have life-threatening experiences without such features (Noyes 1976), while some others have NDE-type experiences when not expecting death at all.

In five subjects in our survey who had near-death experiences during meditation or simple relaxation, while there was a strong sense of impending doom, with one subject claiming that his heart had actually stopped beating, in none of these cases was there any clear physical precipitant or indication of preexisting illness. Four out of five of them heard noises in the early stages, two had a tunnel experience, three saw nonphysical beings—in one case these were beings close to him that had already died—and one subject had a bright light experience. Four out of five of the subjects felt that they were located in the same environment as the physical body. All subjects considered the experience to be of lasting benefit, with four-fifths of them feeling that their life had been changed by this spiritual experience. Thus, these "near-death" subjects had the classical features of the near-death experience as described in Chapter Seven and came close to fulfilling the criteria for Ring's

(1980) sequential NDE stages apparently without being near death at all!

An example of just such an NDE-type OBE occurred in Ms. O., a Jungian therapist who was 49 years old and in excellent health at the time of her experience. She was under "emotional stress at the time, that was letting up." On the night in question she had wished to pursue a fantasy revolving around the Jungian animus archetype. Instead of seeing a male image as expected, after one quite stressful hour she had the following experience:

> I found myself rushing through a tunnel as if pulled by a pneumatic device, or a magnet. It was very fast, but I was aware of a number of small 'doors' on the right hand side, as the tunnel curved left, and that if I were to lose momentum or stop, I would go through one of them, which meant death. It was very frightening, in retrospect, but at the time, was only a matter-of-fact awareness. Then I was literally spewed out into a place of light, and a huge female figure, on a golden throne, looked down at me. I was aware that I had expected a masculine figure, but the momentousness of the occasion lessened that wish. She did not move, except for her eyes, and held, somehow, a number of ropes of light, like neon tubing. My impression was that she was a kind of dynamo, or transformer. Later, I discovered that primitive people have sometimes 'seen' the eyes of divine statues move in the way I saw this figure's eyes move to SEE me. This Seeing was very much like a judgment. My experience was not a recap of my life, but a sense that I had failed to do all I could. I began to say that I was sorry, but the eyes indicated that this did not matter, that she understood and loved me despite the failures. It was an amazing experience of 'Unconditional Love' that I was later to encounter in Buddhist literature. I was about the size of one of the statue's toes.
>
>   An incalculable amount of time went by during the 'visit,' but it became obvious that I should leave, returning through the tunnel, and I worried about the 'doors of death' that I had passed, feeling that I did not have the momentum necessary to be pulled back into wherever I should be. Then I drifted, and became aware that I was dreaming. There was a great sense of relief as I distinguished the dream from that

other state, and realized that the dream state was the entryway—not to the unconscious, but back to consciousness—that it was a journey that I could not manage through my own will alone. Perhaps this makes sense.

Then I slept and woke up in the morning, with a vivid and frightening, but very solemn memory. I have never tried to duplicate this experience, nor felt that it would be necessary. Needless to say, this has transformed my life much as a 'near death' experience might, and my subsequent training and work with schizophrenia is one result.

This account clearly demonstrates how NDE features may occur in subjects who are not near death. Moreover, Jungian psychology places great emphasis on the task of individuation at midlife, and, in fact, Ms. O. experienced just such an existential transformation. In Chapter Nine we will review examples of NDEs from children where the being of light is characterized by us as a forerunner of the developing superego and ego ideal with both punitive, critical, and benign, loving elements. These qualities are clearly depicted in this account as well. The example also illustrates the subjective "feel" of the difference between a dream and the out-of-body state that we discussed in more detail in Chapter Six. Expectancy factors might explain some of the NDE features, although this subject had her experience before the explosion of popular interest in the NDE. Specifically, she claims that it was several years later that she read material that caused her to characterize the experience as an NDE.

After beginning the chapter with an exception, that is, an example in which the subject was not near death, we now return to the rule, that is, the more usual context of the NDE—life-threatening situations. To reiterate the point we made at the end of the last chapter, while NDE features may occur in OBEs not associated with life-threatening illness or injury, they are much more common in the context of a brush with death. Hence, we will devote the major portion of this chapter to those contexts.

In our study circumscribed preexisting factors at the time of NDE include toxic-metabolic, physical injury, illness, psychological set and personality characteristics, and demographic/cultural features, a number of which might, from a commonsense point of view, be thought to affect the intrinsic nature of the experience. This chapter investigates how the context in which the NDE occurs influences the experience itself.

The role of suffering in the near-death experience is as old as Western philosophy itself. In *The Republic*, Plato places great emphasis on the role of death in human development. In the story of Er (*Republic*, pp. 614-21), an ordinary soldier, who suffers a near-fatal injury on the battlefield, is revived on the funeral pyre to describe an experience that contains most of the features reported in near-death experiences. Er's NDE involved journeying with earthly beings from a "dark place to a lighter place," where there were openings in the sky, with further beings guiding him, a moment of judgment, several moments of peace, a quest toward heaven, feelings of joy, weeping, lamenting, and visions of extraordinary beauty and happiness. Plato goes on to describe a complex "light that chains heaven" and holds together the circumference of the sky. The metaphor in the dialogue places emphasis on wisdom that derives from dealing with death, which made an ordinary soldier into a philosophical hero, an experience shared by our subjects, who felt the NDE to be life-changing (Gabbard et al. 1981).

Green (1968) notes in her sample of approximately 400 persons, a majority of whom suffered stress such as illness or accident prior to their out-of-body experiences, that many reported having an unusually wide range of information available to them in this near-death state. In particular many felt that they were able to visit any point of space at will, as did Er. The cities of light that Er described were incorporated at many points in Plato's discussions so as to form an integral part of the foundation for his whole philosophy.

As Stevenson and Greyson (1979) note, if we are to advance in understanding the physiological conditions that accompany and may induce the more impressive subjective experiences, a more careful study of preexisting conditions must be made, thus enabling a determination of what, if any of these features, are determined by the precipitating agent itself. For example cardiac arrest has a final common pathway of physiological effects due to anoxia that, however, produces vastly different reports of these experiences in various resuscitated individuals. Dobson (1971) reports 20 patients, only one of whom remembered a transcendental or mystical type of experience before resuscitation, but in a series by Druss and Kornfield (1967) three of ten survivors of cardiac arrests believed they had entered some unearthly realm or unusual state of consciousness before resuscitation. In a study of seven suicide survivors by Rosen (1975), none reported the panoramic life review, whereas in the series of Noyes and Kletti (1977) 44 percent of the respondents reported such a life review. Only 12 percent of this latter group, however, did not believe they were going to die. Siegel (1980), as we mentioned in the last chapter, places great emphasis on the similarity to hallucinations of the near-death experience and emphasizes many of the physiological preconditions, such as anesthesia, to explain the phenomenological features of the experience. In the study by Sabom (1982), the NDE demonstrated no significant variation between participant groups on a number of demographic and other features such as type of near-death crisis, duration of unconsciousness, and method of resuscitation. Rodin (1980) differs markedly from Sabom's position. He stresses the "commonly held beliefs" amongst groups of individuals and the similarity to a "toxic psychosis."

Three recent surveys of the prevalance and phenomenology of near-death experiences (Lindley 1981; Gallup 1982; Green and Friedman 1983) have included remarkably little information on conditions existing at the time of the NDE. Gallup indicates that in only 60 percent of his cases was there a "description of serious illness, accident, and so on." Unfortunately, although he obtained many opinions regarding people's beliefs about what happens after death, the material he provides on "entrances to eternity" (preexisting conditions) is scanty at best. His cryptic impression was, however, that there were several conditions: 1) physical accidents, where he evokes an explanation based on the view that the threat of danger causes a person to react quickly and effectively to avert serious injury; 2) childbirth, where he emphasizes the anticipation of pain; 3) hospitalizations, operations, and illnesses involving drugs or anesthetics, where he believes firmly that the drugs themselves "may have caused a seemingly supernatural experience"; 4) illness outside of hospitals where the out-of-body aspect of the experience was prominent, and which he suggests may have occurred in as many as two million Americans; 5) criminal attacks, where he implies that the personal attack itself stimulates the mystical experience in an unspecified way; and 6) finally, he mentions a group who are not near death, but who have phenomenologically identical religious visions, dreams, or other spiritual quasi-near-death experiences.

Lindley (1981) reports that 62 percent of his sample were women, a finding similar to our results and to those of Greyson (1980). Lindley believes the female sex domination is due to sampling error, that is, he thinks women are more likely to respond to advertisements. The incidence of accidents in women (52 percent) was much higher than in men (20 percent), whereas near-death experiences due to suicide and illness were approximately equal. In the study by Green (1983), 63 percent of the sample were women, with illnesses and accidents accounting for all but four of the experiences. The other four were suicide attempts.

Although many such accounts are not rigorously controlled, not all of the differences appear attributable to differences in interview technique, use of leading questions, and poor data collection methods. Let us now turn to a careful examination of the preexisting conditions present in our sample.

PREEXISTING CONDITIONS IN 34 NEAR-DEATH EXPERIENCERS

Both univariate and multivariate statistical analyses were performed on our data. We will discuss the former first. Univariate, independent group t-tests were used to examine differences within the NDE group. As independent variables, we used the following conditions: 1) the existence of severe pain, 2) accident, 3) use of drugs, 4) general anesthesia, 5) presence of fever, and 6) cardiac arrest. For this particular section of the analysis, dependent variables included all demographic, phenomenological, and impact items in the POBE and the psychological-test scales. All PAL psychological health items were also included. Corrections were made for heterogeneous variation within the sample, and a probability of 0.05 or better was required for inclusion in this report.

1. *Demographic factors*. At the time of answering our questionnaire, the mean age of the population was 48 years, with a range of 12 through 76 years. Participants reported a mean age at the time of NDE of 28 years, with a range of 3.5 to 60 years. There was no significant clustering of age groups associated with a greater incidence of NDEs. Sixty-five percent of the sample were female, and at the time of the NDE, 51 percent were married, 24 percent single, and 25 percent separated, widowed, or divorced. A wide range of occupational groups was represented, from unemployed individuals to doctoral level professionals; 19.8 percent of the sample were housewives, 7.8 percent were students, and 16.7 percent professionals. Eighteen percent of the sample had completed less than high school education at the time of the study, 17 percent were high school graduates, 35 percent had some college education, 20 percent were college gradu-

ates, and 6 percent had advanced degrees. The general educational level of the population exceeded the 1970 U.S. population census.

Religious background and religious affiliation following the NDE were examined for this population. There were marked changes in religious affiliation before and after the NDE. Those with Protestant backgrounds comprised 65 percent of the sample before NDE and only 48 percent after the NDE. Those with Roman Catholic backgrounds included 19 percent of the sample before NDE and 9 percent of the sample after NDE. Thirteen percent of the sample had a variety of unusual or Eastern religious faiths before NDE and 26 percent after. Three percent of the sample indicated no religious affiliation, rising to 6 percent after the NDE.

Prior interest in mystical experiences or altered states of consciousness was examined because of its obvious potential contribution to the phenomenology of the experience. Thus, experimentation with drugs at any time in the past was questioned. This inquiry covered narcotics, alcohol, minor tranquilizers, amphetamines, psychedelic drugs, and marijuana derivatives. In general drug usage was very low in this population. Seventy-five percent had never used marijuana; 89 percent had never used any psychedelic drugs; and 51 percent reported never having used any other category of drugs. Respondents who were near death actually attended workshops on OBE and mystical experiences significantly less frequently than non-near-death respondents (dF=322, $p<.04$). Forty-four percent of the population had never been hypnotized, while 12 percent had been hypnotized more than 12 times.

2. *Preexisting conditions.* Specific medical conditions existing at the time of the NDE were examined, revealing that 27.6 percent of the sample had a variety of medical illnesses, ranging from viral pneumonia through diabetic coma. Seventeen percent of the sample had their experience while undergoing surgery, which again showed a wide variation of procedures, from minor surgery to cardiovascular operations. Fourteen percent of the sample experienced an NDE during childbirth, one of them during an eclamptic convulsion. Drug intoxication included a variety of mood-altering drugs, including Talwin, LSD, and narcotics, involving 24.5 percent of the sample. In addition 17.5 percent suffered an accident with physical injury, covering a variety of situations from electrocution through drowning. Thirteen participants (38 percent of the sample) had apparently suffered a cardiac arrest prior to the NDE and had been told by medical personnel that their hearts had stopped beating. Sex differ-

ences were also present. Ninety-two percent of females with NDE had their experiences during medical illness compared with only 57 percent of the males. Male respondents tended to have their NDEs more often as a result of accident or physical injury than female respondents, in contrast to the findings of Lindley (1981).

Tables 8.1 through 8.3 summarize the statistical findings.

3. *Psychological health.* Preexisting psychopathology could conceivably affect the experiential aspects of the NDE, as well as its impact. Within the limits of the questionnaire method, attempts were made to assess the mental health of the NDE group from the two perspectives described, that is, the use of the five psychological test scales and the multiscale assessment of psychological health using the PAL scale (see Chapter Two).

As a whole group, the NDE subjects were significantly healthier on PAL items than a group of psychiatric inpatients and outpatients and somewhat healthier than a group of college students. The group differed from the OBE group on only one of the psychological-test scales, the "Absorption" scale. Here the NDE group tended to be more "absorbed" than the OBE group by univariate, independent group t-test ($dF=322$, $p<0.03$). When similarly analyzed using preexisting conditions as the independent variables, those who were under the influence of drugs at the time of the NDE were significantly more "absorbed" ($dF=14$, $p<0.04$) than the other subgroups, while those in severe pain were less hysterical ($dF=7$, $p<0.05$).

Turning now to our multivariate analysis, we used the following 19 variables: At the time of your NDE were you 1) running a high fever, 2) told that your heart had actually stopped beating, 3) under any emotional stress, 4) unusually fatigued, 5) under the influence of alcohol, 6) under the influence of any drug, 7) under general anesthetic, 8) giving birth to a child, 9) in an accident, 10) in severe pain, 11) in a state of physical relaxation, 12) meditating, 13) in a state of mental calmness, 14) dreaming, 15) having a dream involving flying or falling (if dreaming), 16) experiencing sexual orgasm, 17) having an OBE that occurred spontaneously without any effort on your part to leave your body, 18) driving a car or motorcycle, and 19) wanting to have an OBE? Each question was scored "yes" or "no," with room for elaboration in the appropriate places.

THE CONTEXT / 147

Table 8.1
PREEXISTING CONDITIONS: FEVER/CARDIAC ARREST

At the time of your OBE were you running a high fever?
1=Yes, 2=No

Dependent Variable	N	X*	SD	t	dF	P
Heard noises						
Yes	4	1.00	0.00	-2.18	16	0.04
No	14	1.57	0.51			

At the time of your OBE were you told that your heart had actually stopped beating?

Sense of power during OBE						
Yes	13	1.46	0.52	-2.30	29	0.03
No	18	1.83	0.38			
Aware of nonphysical beings who were close, but had already died.						
Yes	10	1.30	0.48	-2.00	24	0.05
No	16	1.69	0.48			

* 1=Yes
  2=No

Table 8.2
PREEXISTING CONDITIONS: DRUG/ANESTHETIC

At the time of OBE were you under the influence of any drug?
1=Yes, 2=No

Dependent Variable	X*	N	SD	t	dF	P
Part of mind or awareness back in physical body.						
Yes	8	2.00	0.00	2.85	31	0.008
No	25	1.48	0.51			
Was a being trying to communicate with you?						
Yes	7	1.00	0.00	-2.52	19	0.02
No	14	1.50	0.52			

Dependent Variable	X*	N	SD	t	dF	P
Awareness of a being of some kind.						
Yes	8	1.00	0.00	−2.01	20	0.05
No	14	1.36	0.49			
Absorption score						
Under influence of drugs	3	28.00	1.00	2.47	14	0.04
Not under influence of drugs	14	22.86	8.59			

At time of your OBE were you under general anesthesia?

Want to keep it a secret.						
Yes	10	1.30	0.48	−3.98	32	0.0001
No	24	1.88	0.34			
Saw a brilliant light.						
Yes	10	1.10	0.32	−2.02	30	0.05
No	22	1.45	0.51			

* 1=Yes
  2=No

Table 8.3
PREEXISTING CONDITIONS: ACCIDENT/PAIN

At the time of OBE were you in severe pain? 1=Yes, 2=No

Dependent Variable	N	X*	SD	t	dF	P
Attached to physical body.						
Yes	11	2.00	0.00	3.06	30	0.005
No	21	1.52	0.51			
Felt confused about experience.						
Yes	13	1.46	0.52	−2.63	32	0.01
No	21	1.86	0.36			
Sense of freedom during OBE.						
Yes	11	1.00	0.00	−2.27	30	0.03
No	21	1.33	0.48			
Saw physical body from a distance.						
Yes	13	1.08	0.28	−2.28	31	0.03
No	21	1.38	0.49			

In same environment as physical body.						
Yes	13	1.15	0.38	−2.09	31	0.04
No	20	1.50	0.51			
Hysteroid score						
In pain	2	8.00	2.83	−2.38	7	0.05
Not in pain	7	13.14	2.67			

At the time of OBE were you in an accident?

Did you want to return to your body?						
Yes	6	2.00	0.00	2.47	29	0.02
No	25	1.48	0.51			
Feeling of joy during OBE.						
Yes	6	1.00	0.00	−2.03	30	0.05
No	26	1.42	0.50			

* 1=Yes
  2=No

The technique used to classify the subjects was a multivariate, cluster analysis for category data developed by Friedman and Rubin (1967) and is discussed in detail in a previous paper (Twemlow et al. 1982). The technique is particularly useful when small numbers of subjects and large numbers of variables are used.

Utilizing the Friedman and Rubin multivariate method, five clusters of subjects were derived, and when the relationship among groups was examined, a discernible structure emerged:

1. *Low-stress cluster.* The 16 subjects in this group were characterized by being relaxed and calm, not meditating, not under emotional stress, not on drugs or alcohol, and without any of the characteristics associated with high anxiety or arousal states. The subjects, however, had a seemingly random distribution of physical causes for their near-death experience, such as childbirth, illness, accident, and so on. None were pyrexic. What is characteristic are their calm and relaxed responses to the experience, in spite of physical circumstances that would normally be accompanied by considerable distress.

2. *Emotional stress cluster.* The six subjects in this cluster all

described themselves as under emotional stress. None was calm, relaxed, or meditating. They were not under the influence of alcohol or drugs during the experience. Once again, other physical preconditions, such as childbirth, accident, and so on were seemingly randomly distributed.

3. *Intoxicant cluster.* This group of four subjects all experienced severe emotional stress without any reports of meditating, being relaxed, or feeling calm. Narcotic drugs and/or alcohol were used in all cases at the time of the NDE.

4. *Cardiac arrest cluster.* The four subjects in this group all experienced cardiac arrest. These subjects reported a primarily meditative state of mind, not necessarily described as relaxed or calm, but associated with dreamlike images, especially flying and falling dreams, implying a sense of movement within the experience.

5. *Anesthetic cluster.* The three subjects in this cluster were all under general anesthetic. They described striking distortions in levels of arousal. Specifically, they were under considerable emotional stress, fatigued, but at the same time, paradoxically felt relaxed and calm. The whole experience was dreamlike in quality.

In an attempt to ascertain the explanatory value of these clusters, one-way analysis of variance followed by Newman-Keuls individual mean comparisons were performed for a number of variables. The variables chosen were: age at the time of reporting the experience, age at the time of the first out-of-body experience, "Absorption" score (Tellegen and Atkinson 1974) danger-seeking score (Tellegen and Atkinson 1974), psychoticism score (Eysenck and Eysenck 1968), hysterical tendency score (Caine 1972), and death anxiety score (Dickstein 1972). There were no significant differences among the clusters for age, danger-seeking, psychoticism, hysterical tendencies, death anxiety, or absorption. There were significant differences for age at first out-of-body experience between the "low-stress" cluster (mean age 29.9 years) and the cardiac arrest cluster (mean age 10 years) ($F=2.956$, $df=-32$, $p<.05$).

Inspection of the phenomenological items and those questions concerning the meaning of the NDE to the individual suggests that the intoxicant-cluster subjects have experiences that are quite vivid, even bizarre and with a confused and magical meaning. They are much more like depersonalization with some hallucinatory features (what we refer to in Chapter Seven as a "before-death" experience).

OVERVIEW

Our cases are remarkably similar in demographic characteristics to those reported by Greyson (1980). His cases show a preponderance of women and of Protestants. Moreover, our study is more randomly selected than Greyson's. Although sampling bias might still hold in our population, the possibility that NDEs are more common in women than in men is suggested by these findings. Our respondents are characteristic of the North American population at large, especially in terms of education, occupational affiliation, and psychological health.

There is little, if any, evidence for the existence of psychiatric disorders in our population. None of the individual test scales measuring psychopathology shows a significant difference between the NDE population as a whole and the respondents who had not had NDEs. Since these calculations did control for high interest and expectation of mystical experiences, the reliability and generalizability of the findings are thus increased. The "Absorption" scale has been widely used as a measure of the capacity to alter consciousness in a number of studies of meditation, biofeedback, hypnosis, and other manipulations of internally directed attention (Davidson 1976). For example in Irwin's (1980) study of 21 Australian undergraduate students, using various measures of visual imagery and cognitive style, OBE participants had less vivid imagery than controls, while their "Absorption" ratings were significantly higher than controls. Hence, the finding of an even higher "Absorption" rating among NDE respondents when compared with an OBE population suggests the possibility that cognitive style might predispose to the near-death experience or perhaps to the recall of it. A high score on this test has also been related to hypnotic susceptibility (Palmer 1975), suggesting once more a cognitive style conducive to experiencing altered states of consciousness. While Irwin's population was "mildly more neurotic" than was a control group, this finding was not supported in our population. Future research into the preexisting psychological set for NDE may more fruitfully examine perceptual-cognitive style rather than preexisting psychiatric pathology.

Religious conditioning might, from a commonsense point of view, be related to the vividness and sense of realness of the NDE. As mentioned in Chapter Seven, Ring (1979) concludes that a change in religiousness appears to be an aftereffect of the NDEs. Sabom (1980), however, finds no significant effect of religious affiliation or frequency of church attendance on variation between NDE subjects. Our sample demonstrates some striking changes, especially from more orthodox to less orthodox religious affiliations following NDE, suggesting that orthodox religious affiliation is altered by the NDE experience.

When specific preexisting medical conditions are examined, one striking overall finding is that the physical cause of the NDE does not appear to have a dramatic effect on the phenomenological consistency of the experience across the respondents, thus supporting similar findings by Siegel (1980), Ring (1980), and others. Participants who had suffered cardiac arrests showed significantly increased feelings of power as well as awareness of persons who had already died around them at the time of the experience, when compared with other NDE respondents. A possible psychodynamic understanding of this finding is that the sense of power can be viewed as part of a manic triumph, representing an omnipotent feeling of having transcended death itself. From the perspective of the contributions of Kohut (1971), one might view this feeling as reflective of the emergence of the grandiose self. The existence of beings might represent infantile wishes for merger experiences with parental figures or relatives who had already died. Moreover, this experience may be linked to the "Golden Fantasy" of an ultimate rescuer (Smith 1977), as we will elaborate in Chapter Nine. The cardiac arrest respondents as a whole, of course, had a more intimate experiential knowledge of death than any other NDE respondents. In this sense the infantile wish to triumph over death has been gratified, at least in the unconscious of the subject.

Those under the influence of drugs report communication with beings and little sense of awareness back in the physical body. They were also more "absorbed." This finding suggests that the drug itself may alter the NDE to produce a syndrome more similar to depersonalization with hallucinatory features. Such experiences are commonly referred to in the LSD literature (Grof 1978). Greyson (1980) and Osis and Haraldsson (1977) note that drug intoxication causes an alteration in the sense of time and diminishes the likelihood of an NDE. Our particular sample of drug abusers, when compared with all others, did not show any significant differences in the sense of time nor in the richness and vividness of the experiences. It should be noted, however, that certain drugs, for example, hyoscine, sometimes used in anesthesia, are known to abolish recall and might explain some of the findings reported by others.

The seeing of a brilliant light by the anesthetic group may reflect the dissociative effect of the anesthetic. Sensations of bright lights and sounds are quite common sequelae of a number of general anesthetics, which induce heightened perceptual sensitivity (for example, ether). The desire to keep the phenomenon a secret might represent a fear that others will think the individual is psychotic, although it may further be explained by the fact that the respondents do have an immediate logical explanation (anesthetic) for their unusual sensations and might not feel the need to discuss it any further.

Participants who were in an accident experienced feelings of joy, along with little desire to return to the physical body, as their distinguishing NDE features. Respondents who were in severe pain experienced a sense of freedom, a visual perception of the physical body from a distance, a sense of not being attached to the body, and an awareness that the body was in the same environment. In this situation the observing self is watching the functioning self being severely damaged, similar to features of depersonalization. Joy and freedom might represent wish fulfillment, an attempt to deny the vulnerability of the physical body as a defense against real physical destruction of the split-off functioning self. In hypnotic pain experiments, it is a common suggestion to dissociate the painful part from the body so that it is treated as "not self" (Schwarz 1979).

In conclusion it seems apparent from our analyses of the data that demographic/cultural variables exert little direct influence on the experience. The impact of the NDE can be marked, however, as indicated by the change in religious affiliation. There is little evidence that an interest in unusual phenomena has direct influence on the nature of the experience itself. While there seem to be no substantial signs of serious psychopathology in the population, there is an indication of a different cognitive-perceptual style in those prone to near-death experiences. Specific medical conditions do appear to affect the nature of the experience, although not markedly. The group of experiences that could be called "before-death" (accident, illness, drug anesthetic, and fever) are much more like depersonalization from the point of view of clinical features than those remembered "after death" (cardiac arrest), which are much more like out-of-body experiences than depersonalization.

Nine — THREE CASE REPORTS OF NEAR-DEATH EXPERIENCE IN CHILDREN

Reports of near-death experiences in small children have only recently begun to appear in the literature. In this chapter we will present two such case reports in children under five and one case report of a slightly older child. The phenomenology of these experiences and their relation to adult cases present us with some fascinating implications.

CASE 1—TODD

Todd was two years, five months old when he bit into the electrical cord from a vacuum cleaner while playing with his siblings. His mother came upon him some two to three minutes after the accident occurred. He was lying motionless, and she initially thought that he might be sleeping. She noted a slightly bluish quality to his skin and instantly became alarmed. Leaning over him, she realized he was not breathing, and she called an ambulance. While awaiting its arrival, she initiated cardiopulmonary resuscitation. She had no formal training in such resuscitative techniques, and she felt wholly inadequate at what she was doing. The ambulance came in approximately seven minutes. The attendants immediately instituted closed cardiac massage, and the child was rushed to the emergency room. An electrocardiogram revealed that the patient was in ventricular asystole with no respiration. Emergency procedures included intravenous sodium bicarbonate to a total of about 30 cc's, intracardiac epinephrine, intracardiac calcium, intravenous calcium, and intubation with artificial ventilation. After a period of time, the cardiac monitor began to reveal activity, but the child went through a further period of ventricular asystole followed by ventricular fibrillation. After two electrical defibrillations, a good cardiac rate and good blood pressure were restored.

Medical records from the hospital emergency room indicate that there was a period of approximately twenty-five minutes when the child had no heartbeat and no respirations. These records also indicate that his pupils were dilated, and that Todd was completely unresponsive on arrival to the emergency room. After spontaneous respirations and heartbeat were reestablished, the patient was transferred to a ward of the hospital where an initial acidosis was quickly corrected with intravenous bicarbonate. Electrolytes, pH and blood gas studies quickly returned to normal that evening. A neurologist was immediately consulted, and when he first examined the patient, he noted that the child was "out of contact," showing irritable crying at times, typical of a thalamic syndrome. There was no evidence of any conscious responses, and there were no responses to visual stimuli. However, he noted that the pupils were equal and reacted well to light. Although occasional movement of the legs occurred, all of the reflexes were suppressed. He started Todd on Decadron intramuscularly. Although the child was initially fed by mouth through reflex action, he did not do well. A nasogastric tube was placed, and Todd was maintained on tube feedings.

After several days of maintenance in this way, there was still no evidence of any response to visual stimuli, despite the fact that the pupils still reacted well, indicating a cortical type of blindness. An EEG showed 4-6 per second, cortical slow rhythms, and was diffusely abnormal with no focal paroxysmal disturbances. Hence, the patient was suffering from a severe encephalopathy related to the anoxia secondary to the cardiac arrest. The result was that the child was in a decorticated state, with marked quadriparesis, apparent blindness, and no evidence of conscious perception.

Over a period of four to six months, Todd gradually regained much of his cortical and neurological functions. He could see again, he could walk, and after about four months, could speak in sentences. No residual mental retardation was present. About three months before his third birthday, he was playing in the living room when his mother asked him, "Could you tell Mommy what you remember when you bit the cord of the vacuum cleaner?" Without even looking up, he told her, "I went in a room with a very nice man and sat with him." His mother asked him what the room looked like. Todd replied, "It had a big bright light in the ceiling," which the mother took to mean some kind of chandelier. Todd's mother then asked him what the man said to him, and Todd responded, "He asked me if I wanted to stay there or come back to you." Looking up at his mother, he said, "I wanted to be with you and come home." Then he smiled and went back to his toys. His mother wrote down these details immediately in his baby book because she was so fascinated by what she had heard. She had never heard of near-death experiences at that time, as this event occurred in 1972, several years prior to the publication of Moody's book.

CASE 2—MIKE

Mike had just turned four years old, when his parents took him to the public swimming pool one hot July day. Mike's mother left him sitting by the edge of the shallow end of the swimming pool, where the water was about three feet deep. She asked her neighbor to watch Mike while she went for a swim. Mike's mother walked about halfway up the Olympic-sized pool and dove in. She looked down at the shallow end and saw that no one was watching Mike. She saw him standing up by the edge of the pool, and then gasped as she saw him squat to look into the pool and fall in head first. She could see his feet sticking out of the water as she frantically swam half the length of the pool to get to him. She estimates that he was submerged between one and two minutes. Finally, just as she got to him, his head surfaced of its own accord. His eyes were huge, larger than she had ever seen them. He looked stunned, but he also looked euphoric. He was a white, ghostly color, but he said he was fine and was neither coughing nor choking.

As she pulled Mike out of the pool, he tried to kick her away, saying he did not want to come out. He said he had seen a long bridge with beautiful, sparkling orange "points" on it, just like Cinderella's Castle at Disneyland. He kept saying that he wanted to go back into the water to see the pretty points again. He also talked of golden lights and pretty colors that he had seen. He excitedly told everyone around the edge of the pool that he had learned to swim and had seen sparkling lights. For one hour he talked about the incident to every passerby. There was not a trace of fear—only euphoria about having learned to swim and about having seen the sparkling points. He had been to Disneyland quite recently, so that he seemed to use Cinderella's Castle as a frame of reference from which to identify the bridge and the lights. After they drove him home from the pool, Mike continued to talk about the lights all day long. He kept saying that he wanted to go back to the pool to see them.

Mike's mother called the pediatrician shortly after they arrived home. He reassured her that he had probably simply hit his head on the bottom of the pool, although there were absolutely no signs of injury on his head. The pediatrician also suggested that Mike had not had enough oxygen during the time he was submerged and was simply hallucinating. When he went to bed that night, Mike woke up in the middle of the night and again mentioned his experience spontaneously to his mother and told her of his wish to go back into the pool to see the brilliant sparkling lights. When he woke up the next morning, again the first thing he said was that he wanted to go back to see the lights. For the ensuing two months, he referred to the experience approximately once a week. Also, for the first few days after his near-death experience, he was very peaceful and talked in a calm, serene way that his mother had never seen before. Mike's mother mentioned that ever since the accident, Mike has loved water and has had no fear of it.

Approximately seven months after the incident, Mike's mother asked him again what he remembered. He said that he remembered the pretty golden lights, but he also said that he remembered an "olden-days cabin" down at the bottom of the golden lights. He said there was a cranky old man in the cabin who didn't say anything. There was no other change in his behavior after the incident.

Mike was a healthy boy who had had no mental, emotional, or physical problems. Neither he nor his mother knew anything about near-death experiences at the time the incident occurred. The family had no religious affiliation.

CASE 3—GAIL

Gail was approximately 29 years old when she was watching a television program in which Dr. Elizabeth Kubler-Ross was discussing the tunnel experience associated with near-death experiences. This was the first she had ever heard of such experiences and led her to share with her mother that she had experienced exactly the same thing as a child. Although it was approximately 22 years later, she remembered it with vivid clarity. She was "deathly ill" and delirious with a complicated case of the mumps. She felt that her body could not recover from the illness, and in desperation she prayed to God. While awaiting death, she heard a soft sound, barely audible. As she continued to listen, she recognized it as being the most beautiful sound she had ever heard in her life. It sounded like a huge chorus of beautiful soprano voices, like angels singing a capella ever so softly. The volume would slowly increase and decrease as she would slip in and out of delirium.

Suddenly, her mind was not only free from the confusion of the delirium, but it was extremely aware of everything around. She felt total peace, complete weightlessness, and absolute freedom. This experience was like nothing she had ever felt before. She found herself floating above her physical body. She could see that she had two separate and distinct bodies in different positions. Her physical body was sleeping, while her other body was hovering over it, wide awake. As she drifted toward the foot of the bed, she saw her mother sitting by the bed crying. Her mother was placing a cloth on the forehead of the sleeping physical body. Despite the fact that her mother was crying, Gail felt detached from the situation and still overwhelmed by peace and joy.

There were other beings in the room with her, appearing as stars or sparks of light that floated all around her. She sensed their presence and mutually peaceful feelings. Then she slowly floated higher away from them until she reached the corner of the ceiling, where she seemed to "bob" softly as she touched the ceiling. She tried to push her hand and arm through the ceiling, and they went right through the ceiling with some slight friction. The next thing she remembered was blackness at the beginning of a tunnel. It was so dark that her eyes were useless, so she simply closed her eyes and enjoyed the exhilarating feeling of movement through the tunnel. She could hear the rushing sound of wind against her body as she was being magnetically drawn or pulled through the tunnel while still floating. As she picked up speed, the sound of the wind became louder, and the exhilarating feeling became greater.

As she gradually began to approach the end of the tunnel, she noted that she could begin to see again. At the end she saw tiny, bright pinpoints of light. She was traveling rapidly toward the light, which became wider and brighter. She was moving so incredibly fast that she was concerned about hitting the sides of the tunnel. She also wondered if she would "crash land" when she reached the end, but instead she stopped abruptly with a soft bounce and was in the presence of a very bright light that made her eyes useless once again.

At that moment a bearded man, about 30 years old, wearing a long white robe appeared to her. She took him to be Christ. He was standing just outside the tunnel, and she could see a beautiful new world beyond the end of the tunnel. She asked the Christ figure if she could go and play in this beautiful new place. She was thrilled when he gave her permission.

She walked down the path past the Christ figure and saw the most beautiful flower garden she had ever seen. The colors were breathtaking and a crystal-clear blue lake was equally beautiful on the other side of the path. Never had Gail seen such a beautiful, pure, and bright setting. She noticed a group of four people, actually two couples, standing on the right of the path and admiring the garden. They were laughing and chatting, and they smiled at her as she approached. She knew instantly that they loved children. She felt immediately accepted, important, loved, and welcomed. She could do no wrong as far as they were concerned, and she was the center of attention.

She continued down the path and stopped and talked with each of several small groups along the way. As she continued, each group of people seemed to become less and less friendly. They began ignoring her, and she felt as though they could not hear her. She was beginning to feel unwelcome. The last person with whom she tried to communicate was rude and totally ignored her. She kept asking him for directions back to the tunnel, but he would not answer her or even acknowledge her presence. It was as though he did not hear her and did not know she was there.

She felt she could find her own way back to the tunnel by following the path backwards. She passed the same people on the way back to the tunnel until she reached the entrance and complained to the Christ figure that some of the people would not talk with her. He smiled a knowing, fatherly smile and said, "It is time to go home." She obediently entered the tunnel and returned to her physical body in the same way she left it.

SIMILARITIES TO ADULT NDES

One of the most striking aspects of these three case reports is the phenomenological similarity between adult and childhood NDEs. At least ten elements in these three case reports are clearly analogous to the adult experiences. 1) In all three cases the phenomenon of the bright light or lights is present. 2) In cases 1 and 3 a loving figure is associated with the light, as in the adult experiences. It is notable that in case 2, the figure is a "cranky old man." Developmental and psychological considerations undoubtedly come into play in the perception of this figure, and we will discuss this aspect of the childhood NDE at greater length later in this chapter. 3) The phenomenon of a border or barrier is present in case 2 in the form of a bridge. 4) The decision of either staying with the light and the figure or returning to one's body is presented in case 1 and case 3, just as in adult experiences. 5) The elation, the sense of peace, and the longing to return to the light characteristic of Mike in case 2 resemble the aftereffects of NDEs reported by adults. 6) The sense of absolute peace, harmony, and freedom reported by Gail in case 3 are typical of feelings reported by adults. 7) Gail's out-of-body experience, in which she experienced herself floating above her physical body that she could see below her, is certainly similar to the adult experience. 8) The sense that there are disembodied beings with her, other than the figure associated with the light, is mentioned in Gail's experience, and is a commonly reported feature of the NDE in adults. 9) The long tunnel reported by Gail in case 3 is also one of the cardinal features of adult NDEs. 10) Finally, the sensation of returning to one's physical body experienced by Gail is commonly experienced in adult NDEs.

As this book goes to press, there are only two reports of near-death experiences in children in the scientific literature (Morse 1983; Bush 1984). Nancy Evans Bush, of The International Association for Near-Death Studies in Storrs, Connecticut, reports 17 cases of childhood NDEs. Fifteen of these are retrospective, as is our case 3, while two are from children under five. Her cases confirm that the pattern of childhood NDEs is similar to that of adult experiences. She noted a similarity to our case 1 in that a three-and-one-half year old also had the experience of sitting with a kind, loving man during his NDE. She also found that the adult element consistently missing from the NDEs of children was the kaleidoscopic review of one's life, often referred to as panoramic memory. This finding raises the possibility that the panoramic memory feature is at least partly a function of chronological age.

The other report of a near-death experience in a child found in the scientific literature comes from Morse (1983), a pediatrician who treated a seven-year-old female child in the emergency room following a near-drowning event. Although she was initially comatose with fixed and dilated pupils, she was successfully resuscitated with little residual damage. One week subsequent to the accident, she related her near-death experience. She was aware that she was dead and was traveling through a tunnel, accompanied by a female guide. The tunnel became very bright, and she felt that she was going to heaven. She described heaven as "fun. It was bright and there were lots of flowers." She also described a border around which she could not see, and she met a number of people, including dead grandparents and a dead maternal aunt. A loving figure was present, whom she identified as "Heavenly Father and Jesus," and this figure asked her if she wished to return to earth. When she replied, "No," the female guide asked her if she wanted to see her mother. After saying that she did, she woke up in the hospital.

As is evident from the summarized description of the NDE reported by Morse, at least eight of the ten elements analogous to adult experiences are present in this case. The two possible exceptions are the out-of-body experience, as Morse's case does not report seeing herself floating above her physical body and the sensation of returning to her physical body. It is noteworthy that this child also did not report the phenomenon of panoramic memory. The child's mother reported that she wished to go back to the place that she called heaven and frequently asked for people she had met there.

The child came from a deeply religious Mormon background, but Morse notes that although many aspects of her NDE were reminiscent of her religious training, her experience was consistent with adult NDEs in ways that could not be explained by her religious background. For example the phenomenon of the dark tunnel to heaven, the border around heaven, and the choice to return to earth were not included in her religious teachings.

The consistency of the near-death experience in the child has implications for the various explanatory hypotheses discussed in Chapter Eight. Consistent phenomenological features in the NDEs of small children make the cultural programming argument untenable. Todd was two-and-one-half at the time of his experience, and certainly was not influenced by religious teaching or media input. Mike was four and had not heard anything of near-death experiences nor had he been to Sunday School, where he might have been subject to religious teachings. Although one must consider the possibility that the mothers revised the experiences when they reported them to us, neither knew anything about near-death experiences at the time the incident occurred. The three case reports illustrate the repeated finding that while the phenomenology of NDEs is culturally and demographically consistent, the interpretation of the features varies depending on one's experience and one's culture. For example the seven-year-old Gail was able to identify the figure as Christ, which was obviously related to religious teachings and her greater chronological age, when one can place a figure in a certain religious context better than one can at the age of two-and-one-half or four. Whereas adults in the United States typically identify the figure as Christ or God, persons who have had near-death experiences in India typically identify the figure as a well-known yogi (Khemka 1983). Similarly, Mike identifies the border or barrier as a bridge of lights similar to the one he saw at Cinderella's Castle at Disneyland. This interpretation of the feature was, of course, based on Mike's own limited experience. In India the border or barrier is almost always identified as the Ganges River (Khemka 1983). One of the most intriguing and valuable aspects of the study of these childhood experiences is the differences in perception of the being of light connected with the NDE.

BEING OF LIGHT

In considering the nature and meaning of the being of light, it must first be stated that this figure is variously perceived by different NDEers, whether adult or child. Some see a figure separate from the light, a figure with discernible features, enabling the individual to identify the figure as Christ or a familiar yogi. Others see the light itself as a being without discernible face or body. Still others see no being, only a brilliant light and an overwhelming sense of love and acceptance. The subjects who see no being in the light may nevertheless see other figures accompanying them to the light, who may or may not speak to them. These figures are often deceased relatives. The unearthly and extraordinary sense of love and peace often attracts the individual to stay with the light rather than to return. There is ordinarily some sort of communication with the being of light, although not verbally. In some of Moody's cases (1975), the figure in the light asks the NDEer if he or she loved while on earth. Occasionally, the panoramic replay of one's life history is accompanied by highlighting those instances in one's life when one clearly expressed love toward others. This sense of benign judgment is ordinarily accompanied by a command to go back and finish what one had set out to do. The figure associated with the light may also offer the NDEer a choice of whether he or she would prefer to stay or to return to his or her body.

Just as the interpretations of the identity of the figure associated with the light depend on one's individual and cultural past, so do the qualities attributed to significant figures in one's current life reflect qualities from important figures in one's past. From the psychoanalytic viewpoint, all significant objects (persons) in one's life are transference objects to one degree or another. In other words the way another person is perceived is partly a function of the perceiver's attributing qualities of persons from his or her own past to the perceived person. The process of child development is one of internalizing parental qualities and forging one's identity out of this smithy of internalized objects and their qualities. By the time the normal child is three years of age, he or she has attained object constancy, which is the ability to soothe oneself with the internal, emotionally charged image of one's mother during times of her absence.

When the child traverses the oedipal phase of development, between the ages of roughly three and seven, the superego and ego ideal are formed from these internalized parental objects. Subsequently, the individual experiences others more like the projected images of one's own internal objects.

Given the pervasive nature of transference in all human interactions, it is reasonable to assume that the way any significant figure, such as the being of light during the near-death experience, is perceived reflects something about the internal objects of the NDEer. Indeed, many accounts of the being of light are reminiscent of superego and ego ideal functions, that is, proscriptions and prescriptions stemming from parental attitudes, which have been internalized and made one's own. The NDEer experiences the figure as giving him or her loving acceptance as well as benign judgment and a command to return. As Sandler (1960) has indicated, self-esteem and superego are very much related in that the child can restore his or her original state of well-being by two methods: 1) obedience to and compliance with the demands of the parents, and 2) identification with the parents. Schafer (1960) writes of "the loving and beloved superego," pointing out that the superego in Freud's model is far more than a critic of one's behavior. As the internalized parent, the superego also provides protection and comfort, ideals and pride, and adaptation to the parental superego. At times when the survival of the organism is threatened, the individual strives to maintain self-esteem and to soothe the overwhelming anxiety accompanying the prospect of imminent death. These internalized parental qualities, which are referred to as the superego and ego ideal in Freud's structural model, may come to the rescue in the form of the being of light. The individual feels loved, protected, and comforted. Further confirmation of this viewpoint comes from the fact that sometimes the beings viewed during the near-death experience are the subject's deceased parents, expressing their love and longing for the NDEer, as well as often urging him or her to return and take care of his or her affairs on earth. Moreover, the panoramic replay of one's life is often associated with a sense of having been purged of accumulated guilt feelings.

Yalom (1980) notes that most of us harbor omnipotent fantasies of triumph over death in two forms, which may be stated in the first person as follows: 1) "It will always be someone else who dies, not me"; and 2) "Someone will ultimately rescue me from death." This second notion of the ultimate rescuer has been elegantly developed by Smith (1977), who terms this fantasy the "Golden Fantasy." In Smith's view the fantasy of the ultimate rescuer is a universal one that shapes our behavior, our fantasy lives, and our relations to others. He found in psychoanalytic work with a number of patients of varying diagnoses and ego strengths a consistent wish to have all of one's needs met in a relationship hallowed by perfection. The fantasy is always a passive one wherein there is a conviction that one will be rescued from despair by a fantasied and ill-defined person somewhere in the universe who is fully capable of meeting one's needs. The developmental origins of this fantasy are probably related to the infant's experience that mother is always there when he or she needs her, as though he or she had omnipotent control over her every move. Furthermore, in Smith's words, the individual may have, "The subjective experience...that this fantasy touches on the deepest issues of one's life and that indeed one's very survival may depend on its preservation" (p. 311). One can infer that this fantasy serves as one defense against the existential despair associated with the certainty of extinction at death. The trauma of a life-threatening crisis may activate this repressed and regressive infantile wish to be reunited with a loving parent, who will rescue the NDEer.

This psychoanalytic discussion of the nature of transference objects, superego and ego ideal information, and internalized object relations lead us directly into a consideration of NDEs in children. Detailed study of the near-death experience in children allows us to catch a glimpse of the development of internalized object relations and superego formation in childhood. For example, in Todd's experience, the figure associated with the light is an all-good, loving figure, who simply offers Todd a choice as to whether he would like to return or stay. There is no judgment passed and no command issued. Mike's experience is of a "cranky old man" in a cabin. This figure is also one-dimensional. These two figures lack the richness and complexity of the adult NDE figure. They resemble ordinary, nonmystical parental figures. However, these figures are certainly in keeping with what we would expect of children in preoedipal or early oedipal phases of development. Prior to the development of a full-blown oedipus complex, internalized objects are split into all-good and all-bad. Self-representations are similarly split. The whole object, ambivalently viewed as both good and bad, is an accomplishment of the oedipal period and hence cannot be expected to be present in preoedipal children. The one-dimensional nature of Todd's and Mike's figures is in keeping with their developmental stage.

As we move to case 3, we undertake the examination of Gail, a seven-year-old child who has traversed the oedipal phase of development and is beginning to enter latency. The figures in her near-death experience are much more well formed, although we cannot rule out the possibility that the experience has been significantly revised since it is a retrospective account from an adult. The Christ figure is clearly a loving one, while the other figures around her become less and less loving, until they are rude to the point of ignoring her. In these figures we see both good and bad qualities, although they are still not integrated into one individual. We also sense something of the injured narcissism of the child who fails to get the mirroring or validating responses she seeks (Kohut 1971). In the adult NDE the being of light is closer to a whole object, ambivalently viewed as one would view a parent. This figure loves and accepts the NDEer while judging how the NDEer has lived his or her life and commanding the NDEer to return. This being of light is a well-rounded figure who evokes both love and fear in the subject. It is no coincidence that this figure is often taken to be God, since the Western anthropomorphized view of God is the powerful parent, that is, God, the Father, who evokes both fear and love in his subjects.

To summarize the point we are making about this aspect of NDEs in children, the study of the figures associated with these childhood experiences reflects the developmental level of the child's internalized object relations and of the child's superego formation. This type of study is of considerable value in advancing our knowledge of the nature of the development of moral behavior and internalized object relations in children. To undertake an examination of this type, we run the risk of having our method misconstrued. We are not implying in this analysis that the being of light is definitively the internalized parent of the NDEer. That may or may not be the case. We are saying that whatever figure is perceived in the course of the near-death experience will be perceived through an individual filter or template of internalized objects, which is developmentally determined by the age of the child and the child's experience with significant objects in his or her environment.

This chapter concludes our series of three chapters on the near-death experience. Our intent has been to focus on some unique contributions that we have made to this literature based on our study of out-of-body experiences. Since our psychoanalytic orientation and training are unusual among NDE researchers, it has also been our intent to build bridges between the phenomenology of the near-death experience and the psychoanalytic understanding of the intrapsychic world.

Part IV
UNDERSTANDING THE OUT-OF-BODY EXPERIENCE

Ten — THE METAPSYCHOLOGY OF ALTERED MIND/BODY PERCEPTION

This chapter begins the fourth and final section of our book. Up to this point we have examined a variety of forms of altered mind/body perception and reviewed both our own data and those of others regarding such experiences. It is our intention in this final section to synthesize the various data with the help of psychoanalytic, philosophical, and neurophysiological viewpoints, so that a coherent, multiperspective, theoretical framework can be brought to bear in our efforts to understand these phenomena. We begin this endeavor in the current chapter with metapsychological considerations about the nature of altered mind/body perception. Hinsie and Campbell (1975) define metapsychology as "that branch or extention of psychology which deals with the philosophical significance of mental processes, the nature of the mind/body interrelationship, the origin and purpose of the mind, and similar speculations that are beyond the reach of empirical verification" (p. 469). The breadth of such a definition reflects the debate about the usefulness and meaning of metapsychology that has been raging since the origins of psychoanalysis.

Holt (Chattah 1983) has traced the history of the term. Freud himself gave a diversity of meanings to the word. Metapsychology was initially a depth psychology, which would explain behavior and symptoms according to unconscious conflicts. It was also originally an effort to construct a neurological-biological underpinning of theory that would correlate with psychological data. Freud later delineated metapsychology as a theory separate from the clinical theory. Metapsychology was to be a broader, more explanatory system that approached the ideal of the natural science. Freud made explicit the idea that metapsychology transcended a mere psychology of the unconscious and was intended to clarify theoretical assumptions on which clinical psychoanalysis could be founded. As the term evolved, Freud also used metapsychology to denote a synthetic psychology that bridged psychoanalysis and philosophy. Holt repeatedly emphasizes that metapsychology was intended to be a system distinct from the therapeutic theories gleaned from the consulting room.

To clarify our usage of the term in the context of this chapter, we return to our statement in Chapter One, where we indicated that our primary interest in altered mind/body perception is of a psychological nature. Hence, we are not interested in using the phenomena as a springboard for either metaphysical speculation nor for purely biological explanations. Psychoanalysis is a general psychology applicable to understanding normal mental functioning as well as a clinical therapeutic technique. The topographic, the structural, the dynamic, the economic, and the genetic models of psychoanalysis are not merely tools for explanatory formulations of psychopathological entities; they are also general principles of mental functioning. Our effort here to link phenomena of altered mind/body perception to metapsychological underpinnings is simply an endeavor to understand these experiences in the context of the existing theoretical frameworks by which we understand general intrapsychic functioning. While Freud eschewed the mingling of metapsychology and clinical theory, in actual practice the clinician repeatedly seeks to understand the material presented to him or her in the consulting room by relying on metapsychological constructs. Similarly, we will apply our metapsychological understanding both to normal phenomena and to that considered psychopathological. More specifically, we seek to understand altered mind/body perception in terms of an ego-psychological framework, which leads us to the ideas of Paul Federn.

THE EGO PSYCHOLOGY OF FEDERN

Working in the first half of the twentieth century, Federn developed his theories based on accurate descriptions of the subjective experiences of healthy, as well as diseased persons. While Freud conceptualized the ego as a rather impersonal executive organ that mediated between internal pressures from the id and the superego on the one hand, and external pressures from the environment on the other, Federn viewed the ego in a much more personal way. He insisted that the ego is a subjective experience (1952), that is, one has an actual sensation of one's own ego, which may be called "ego feeling."* He defined ego feeling as, "the feeling of bodily and mental relations in respect to time and content, the relation being regarded as an uninterrupted or a restored unity" (1952, p. 25). More subtly, he refers to it as "the sensation, constantly present, of one's own person—the ego's own perception of itself" (1952, p. 60). The metapsychological basis of this ego feeling is a state of psychical cathexis (investment of mental energy) of certain interdependent bodily and mental functions and contents. The ego feeling fluctuates during the course of a day so that its content is always shifting despite the fact that it is constantly uniting all relations and parts of the ego into a single whole.

Through studies of the dreaming ego, Federn further delineated that the coherent ego unit may be subdivided into a bodily ego and a mental ego. The mental ego is almost always experienced as being inside the bodily ego, and, therefore, the separation of the two components becomes evident only in dreaming or in other special states. They are united in such a way that the bodily ego feels the body to be outside, between the mental ego and the external world. Federn notes that the phrase, "mind and body," actually refers to "mental and bodily ego." It is our thesis that these two subdivisions of the ego feeling commonly separate in experiences of altered mind/body perception, a point to which we will return shortly.

Federn's understanding of ego development put him at odds with some of Freud's views. While Freud asserted that the ego was first and foremost a body ego (1923), Federn believed otherwise. He noted the paradox that the ego is both subject and object simultaneously. The ego is the bearer of consciousness, yet the individual person is also conscious of his or her own ego. In other words there is a reflective part of the ego and another part of the ego that is reflected upon. However, Federn postulated an original and even more primitive form of ego that he termed objectless. He termed this neutral,

---

*We are aware that this experience-near construct would probably be labeled the "self" by Kohut (1971) and by other contemporary psychoanalytic authors. We retain Federn's usage intentionally to avoid further semantic complications.

objectless form of ego cathexis as the "medial ego feeling," using the middle voice of classical Greek to capture the idea that it is neither active nor reflective. This medial ego feeling, as Rinsley (1962) has pointed out, forms the matrix from which self-awareness develops. It predates the elaboration of a body ego and applies to the most primitive, general feeling tone of the infant when he or she is in the earliest undifferentiated stages of development. The cognitive components of this feeling tone have been termed "proto-thoughts" by Bion (Grinberg et al. 1977). Primitive thoughts exist from the beginning, according to Bion, and give rise to the process of thinking, as a way of manipulating these thoughts. By thinking, that is, reflection, the organism is able to unburden the psyche of an overwhelming amount of stimuli. These archaic thoughts begin as mere sense impressions accompanying primitive emotional states, according to Bion, and appear genetically and epistemologically prior to the capacity to think. Rinsley links this primitive state to Sartre's notion of "pre-reflective cogito" (1957), by which he refers to the fact that one somehow knows that one simply is irrespective of one's ability to reflect on one's awareness of one's being.

Hence, the important point here for our discussion is that an ego feeling exists from the earliest days of postnatal existence that predates and is independent of the establishment of a bodily ego feeling. As Rinsley (1962) indicates, this medial ego feeling forms the nexus for the development of a general affect-laden feeling tone, which Federn has termed "buoyancy." At this point the infant does not experience boundaries because the infant has not yet confined his or her conscious awareness to the limitations of his or her physical body. Nor does the infant cathect himself or herself as an object on which reflection is possible. Federn views this early medial component of the ego cathexis as the element responsible for the adult feeling that everyday life is pleasantly familiar rather than empty, disagreeable, and meaningless.

As development proceeds, this pleasant boundariless state is superseded by the development of ego boundaries, another important concept of Federn's theory. Ego boundaries delineate what is "me" from what is "not me," as we discussed in Chapter Five in the context of schizophrenic psychopathology. Ego boundaries apply both to mental boundaries and to body boundaries. Federn viewed the ego boundary as a peripheral sense organ that also discriminated what was real from what was unreal. He repeatedly emphasized that these ego boundaries are quite flexible and at different times, various sensory data or material in external reality could lose its ego cathexis and come to be experienced differently by the individual. Freud himself recognized this phenomenon when he wrote in *Civilization and Its Discontents*: "Pathology has made us acquainted with a great number of states in which the boundary lines between the ego and the external world become uncertain or in which they are drawn incorrectly. There are cases in which parts of a person's own body, even portions of his own mental life—his perceptions, thoughts and feelings—appear alien to him, as not belonging to his ego; there are other cases in which he ascribes to the external world things that clearly originate in his own ego and that ought to be acknowledged by it. Thus, even the feeling of our own ego is subject to disturbances and the boundaries of the ego are not constant" (1930, p. 66).

While in the healthy adult, the bodily ego cathexis and the mental ego cathexis are fused together and firmly integrated in a clearly established ego boundary, fluctuations occur regularly, although we typically do not attend to these fluctuations. A simple example is the fact that when we are driving an automobile, we allow our boundaries to extend and include the automobile so that we have a very clear sense of the proximity of the rear fender to the car behind us. Another common example of a defect in the bodily ego boundary occurs with dental anesthesia, as Federn himself points out (1952). During a dental procedure, Federn had his left mandibular nerve blocked. This anesthesia was experienced as a triangular gap in the left wall of his mouth cavity. His cheeks and lips, when touched by his finger, seemed no longer to belong to the body. His bodily ego was indented, and he could not use his memory of those anatomical structures to fill the defect. This example clearly indicates how the bodily ego boundary is formed by proprioceptions transmitted by sensory nerves along with a cathexis from the ego. One does not feel paralysis of the sensory nerve, simply a vacuum of that location in the body. Such an experience suggests the presence of a mental sensory organ.

While such demonstrations of the flexibility of ego boundaries are commonplace, the notion of dissociation between the bodily ego cathexis and the mental ego cathexis may at first glance seem more controversial. Federn, however, cites three common instances in which this occurs: 1) the dream state, 2) gradual loss of consciousness, such as fainting, and 3) the transition into and out of sleep. Clearly, the out-of-body experience is also a common example of the separation of the mental ego feeling from the bodily ego feeling.

Federn was apparently relatively unfamiliar with this phenomenon and did not investigate it in a thoroughgoing manner. However, he does make a passing reference to such states in describing the dissociation of body ego from mental ego in an attack of fainting: "Here the body ego is felt to slip away from one and slide downwards in the strangest manner; sometimes the distal extremities go before the proximal parts; for a short space of time, the mental ego alone is felt in a definite way, an experience that never occurs under any other conditions. It may be that it accompanies states of ecstasy and is responsible for the self-evident dualistic conviction of the separate existence of body and soul. The ascension-myth is a projected representation of such experiences" (1952, p. 29).

Federn says this dissociation is most evident in dreams, where the bodily ego is typically not felt while the mental ego is involved in dreaming.* The "dream ego" is in such instances the mental ego only. If one is willing to sacrifice the natural process of falling asleep, one can experience the mental ego independent of the bodily ego as one is on the verge of falling asleep. The sensation of the distal parts of the body disappear first, and the bodily ego gradually retreats upward toward the head. As one begins to enter the hypnagogic state, one can experience a nonphysical conscious representation as a "mental ego." Rinsley (1962) notes that some individuals report this representation as a bright, curved spheroidal surface, like an ovoid ball, somewhere in the vicinity of the head. The crucial point to underscore from this observation is that after decathexis of the bodily ego, there yet remains a clearly cathected sense of "self" or "mental ego." This coherent mental ego cathexis is the closest we can come in adult life to experiencing the early medial ego feeling, from which all subsequent ego states derive. However, this mental ego is capable of reflection and, therefore, is not objectless or prereflective. Rinsley points out the neurological analogy of this situation in patients with autotopagnosias and anosagnosias secondary to brain injuries. These patients are unable to experience and may disown certain parts of their bodies, but they still have a clear sense of self.

A summary of the essential notions of Federn that we have been developing in the course of this discussion may be useful at this point. In the postnatal boundariless state of the infant, there is a prereflective self-awareness that is noncorporeal, that is, independent

---

*The classic exception to this observation is the lucid dream (see Chapter Six).

of bodily feeling. This state is followed by the development of the capacity for noncorporeal reflectiveness—the mental ego cathexis. As infants leave the symbiotic stage with their mothers and develop a sense of themselves as separate entities, they develop, through kinesthetic and tactile bodily sensations, a bodily ego cathexis that supersedes and encompasses the original medial ego feeling and its successor, the mental ego cathexis. Ego boundaries, including body boundaries, are elaborated and cathected by the psychic apparatus of the infant. A certain amount of mental energy or cathexis is required to maintain the ego boundary as well as the fusion of the bodily and mental ego feelings. Fluctuations in this cathexis create variations both in the ego boundary and in the fusion of mental and bodily ego feelings so that under certain circumstances, they may be separated. However, as Rinsley (1962) notes, when the mental ego is differentiated from the bodily ego, it has a reflective cathexis, while the original medial ego feeling is from the beginning prereflective. The former is a reflective entity because the individual can clearly attend to it, concentrate on it, or reflect upon it, as opposed to the pure being of the early medial ego feeling. In the mature ego boundary, then, both medial and reflective cathexes reside.

A CONTINUUM OF ALTERED MIND/BODY PERCEPTION

Federn's conceptualization of ego development allows us to postulate a continuum of experiences of altered mind/body perceptions, ranging from the prototypical out-of-body experience at the nonpathological end of this spectrum through depersonalization in the middle of the continuum and finally to the schizophrenic body disturbances at the pathological end of the spectrum. We omit autoscopic phenomena from this continuum because, in our view, this metapsychological framework does not apply to autoscopy. As we indicated in Chapter Four, autoscopy, as defined narrowly, does not involve a true alteration of mind/body perception. The subject identifies his or her double as a phantom and as an hallucination. The subject's mind remains identified with his or her body, which does not undergo distortion. While autoscopic phenomenon may be confused with forms of altered mind/body perception, such as out-of-body experience, depersonalization, or schizophrenic body boundary disturbances, it requires a different set of metapsychological constructs. The visual perception of the phantom is paramount in autoscopy, whereas the subjective sense of spatial dislocation is most important in other forms of altered mind/body perception.

A caveat similar to the one in Chapter Five is indicated, however, as we propose this continuum. Both out-of-body experience and depersonalization may occur in a schizophrenic patient. Schizophrenia is a constellation of symptoms that form a psychiatric syndrome. Depersonalization and out-of-body experience are not. Depersonalization is merely a symptom occurring within a syndrome or as an isolated event in a normal subject. Out-of-body experience is a nonsymptomatic altered state of consciousness, not necessarily confined to normal or abnormal subjects. Although our survey respondents tended to be healthier than the normal population, this finding does not exclude the possibility of an OBE occurring in a psychotic individual.* This continuum is primarily of heuristic value in providing a metapsychological basis by which to understand the variations in the common forms of altered mind/body perception, from ecstatic states of heightened awareness and integration to disorganizing episodes of psychotic decompensation. Furthermore, it is based on the assumption that the OBE is the prototype of altered mind/body perception, a point of reference from which other states deviate, with more or less pathological implications.

In out-of-body experience, there appears to be a withdrawal of cathexis from the bodily ego, while cathexis is maintained in the mental ego. This dissociation of mental from bodily ego is cited by Federn in the process of falling asleep. It is of interest, in this regard, that 80 percent of the subjects of the OBE subjects in our study, reported that their OBE occurred in a state of physical relaxation and mental calmness. Similarly, meditators frequently report out-of-body experiences. Like the individual who is resting or attempting to fall asleep, the meditator is characterized by a state of mental relaxation and physical immobility. To a large extent, the position of the body in space, and therefore the body boundary or bodily ego feeling, is dependent on movement. Motion of the arm through space, for example, lets us know clearly where the arm is through the sensory neural pathways originating in the arm. When the arm is motionless, as it is in passive meditative states, or resting states, one begins to lose track of the sensation of the arm and starts to decathect the arm and the rest of the body, as one's psychic energy and attention is not required. Indeed, meditators commonly report the feeling that the

---

*Such an example will be provided in Chapter Eleven.

distal parts of their extremities are no longer sensed as part of them during meditation. Hence, one can postulate that the dissociation of the mental ego from the bodily ego is more likely to be induced by situations where the body is at rest and requires less psychic energy investment.

Moreover, in the out-of-body experience, an important distinction is that while the body boundary has been decathected, the ego boundary of the individual remains intact. The individual does not experience his or her identity as disturbed in the least. The individual does not experience a fusing with other individuals, as a schizophrenic with disrupted ego boundaries does. Also, the sense of bouyant, positive ego feeling is preserved, as evidenced by the reports of the overwhelming majority of our OBE subjects that the experience was both pleasant and more real than a dream.

Our formulation of the underlying mechanism of out-of-body experience up to this point leaves an important question unanswered: If, in fact, the bodily ego has been decathected in the out-of-body state, why is it that 76 percent of the OBE subjects in our study reported that in the out-of-body state they were in a form similar to the physical body? Clearly, the typical OBE subject must retain to some extent the feeling of his body. A short vignette may be helpful to demonstrate this phenomenon. Dr. P., a 29-year-old professor had returned from a business trip on a Sunday afternoon, when he lay down in bed to take a nap. He reclined on his left side when he got in the bed. This position felt uncomfortable, so he rolled onto his back. Nothing seemed unusual in his new position on his back, until he realized that he was looking at his right shoulder in the position that it had previously occupied when he was lying on his left side. He then started floating upwards toward the ceiling and realized he was having an out-of-body experience. He immediately snapped back into his body when the phone rang. This example illustrates how some sensation of the body was retained, enabling the professor to feel that he had indeed rolled over on his back.

We are thus faced with the paradox that the bodily ego has apparently been decathected, but a feeling of the body remains in the out-of-body state. To understand this paradoxical state of affairs, we turn to the work of Schilder (1935), a pioneer in the elucidation of the mental representation of the body. Schilder introduced the terms body image and body scheme. The body image consists of the proprioceptions of the whole body. It changes with the body's varying movements and postures accordingly. The body scheme represents the constant mental knowledge of one's body. While the body *scheme* is a constant mental configuration, the body image is constantly in flux as the body changes its position and posture. Throughout all these changes, the bodily ego is the continuous awareness of one's body. Hence, image, scheme, and ego are all mental rather than somatic phenomena. However, the bodily ego is not identical with the body image or the body scheme described by Schilder. It is only when the body image is completely invested with bodily ego feeling that there is a one-to-one correspondence between bodily ego and body image. Similarly, as Federn has pointed out, the bodily ego can disappear without involving the somatic organization of the body, which allows for proper use of the body parts. To summarize, the body scheme is a cognitive phenomenon involving the mental representation of the body; the bodily ego refers to the feeling level—it is an affect-laden sense of buoyant awareness of one's body.

As we return to the out-of-body experience and our attempt to apply these constructs to that phenomenon, we can now better understand the observations of the OBE subjects. The out-of-body experience begins when cathexis is withdrawn from the bodily ego feeling and the mental ego cathexis is experienced as separate from the body. Despite this disengagement of the mental ego from the bodily ego, the cognitive body scheme remains elaborated by the mental ego, as it is, after all, a purely mental phenomenon. No sooner has this dissociation of mental ego from bodily ego occurred than the cathexis withdrawn from the bodily ego is secondarily reinvested. This time, however, the cathexis is shifted from the actual body to the body *scheme* elaborated by the mental ego. Hence, the subject in the out-of-body state has the subjective sensation of a body ego feeling. The subject then may move about in his or her out-of-body state and attempt to touch the wall with his or her newly elaborated body, referred to as "astral body" or "etheric body" by parapsychologists and theosophists. When this second body attempts to touch the wall, for example, what is "out" of the body is an engram of touch—a memory trace which is indistinguishable to the subject from the real sense of touch when the subject is "in" the body. The indistinguishable nature of this engram may partially account for the subjectively perceived reality of the experience.

This sensation of having a body in the absence of one seems extraordinary at first glance, but is, in fact, a well-known clinical phenomenon. The phantom limb experience of amputees is directly analagous to what we are describing in the out-of-body state. Following the loss of the limb, the cognitive body scheme of that limb, a purely mental phenomenon, remains and is invested with bodily ego feeling so that the amputee feels that the amputated limb is still there. The amputee may automatically reach down to scratch an itch in the phantom limb. It is not uncommon for the amputee to complain of the persisting sensation of the limb for many years. Mahler and McDevitt (1982) cite phantom limb phenomena as evidence of the primary developmental importance of integrating various part images of the body into a whole self-image. When the integrity of the body image as a whole is threatened, they point out, there is a powerful tendency to employ restitutive mechanisms to restore the sense of a complete and cohesive body. They note the frequent anatomical position responses on the Rorschach tests of phantom limb patients and assert that this finding reflects how the patients are almost continually preoccupied with compensatory efforts to restore the compromised body scheme to its former wholeness. Similarly, an instant restitutive process occurs when the mental ego is disengaged from the bodily ego through the mechanism of cathexis shift from the actual body to the cognitive body scheme. What we witness in the phantom limb phenomenon is what we witness in the out-of-body experience, namely, a body scheme fully cathected with bodily ego feeling without a physical body component.

As we move down the continuum into the realm of depersonalization and derealization, we note some similarities, but the differences are far greater. In this section of the continuum, there is considerable variation. Derealization involves no alteration of the mind/body relationship, but merely the feeling that familiar objects in the environment are strange and unreal. As we noted in Chapter Three, approximately 81 percent of persons experiencing depersonalization do not note frank detachment of the mind from the body. For the sake of this excursion into metapsychology, we will here consider only that 19 percent who do feel a disruption of the mind/body relationship. As in out-of-body experience, the bodily ego cathexis and the mental ego cathexis may be separated, although not invariably as in OBE. However, both the bouyant ego feeling and the intact ego boundary characteristic of out-of-body experience are not present in depersonalization. Federn comments that there is a withdrawal of the libidinal component from the cathexis of the ego boundary in depersonalization so that the experience is empty, strange, and unpleasant. The ego feeling is similarly deficient, and Federn refers to the empty knowledge of one's self typical of depersonalization as mere "ego consciousness" as opposed to ego feeling. These impairments in ego boundaries and ego feeling are also typical of dream states and account for the frequent report of individuals with depersonalization that their depersonalized states are "dreamlike." In the dream the mental and bodily ego cathexes are usually separated since one is aware only of one's psychic processes. We are ordinarily not aware of the absence of the bodily ego in dreams, unlike out-of-body experience, where the subject is quite aware of this deficiency. Federn notes that there is such strict economizing of ego cathexis in dreams that only the bare minimum necessary to experience dream images is utilized. The dream ego, then, is a mere shadow of the normal, buoyant ego of the waking state since only a fraction of the cathexis of the ego boundary is required by the dream image at any given moment. As Freud (1900) observed, dreams are the guardian of sleep; they preserve it rather than disrupt it. Hence, in normal sleep the mental ego awakens as little as possible and the bodily ego does not awaken at all. The dream ego, then, is poorly cathected. Many ego functions, such as reasoning, judgment, and volition are lacking, so that the dream ego is in a compromised position.

The parallels between the "dream ego" and depersonalization episodes are clear. Both have impaired ego feelings and compromised ego boundaries. These factors account for the dreamlike and unpleasant quality inherent in depersonalizing episodes. The ego weaknesses associated with depersonalization may be conducive to its use in the service of primitive defense mechanisms such as splitting, where the observing self detaches itself from the functioning self, to which it attributes unacceptable and disavowed qualities (Gabbard 1979). Similarly, depersonalization episodes may accompany experiences of self-fragmentation in narcissistically disturbed or schizophrenic patients, as described in Chapter Three. In our survey of the many causes of depersonalization in that chapter, none seems particularly specific. Federn notes this fact and comments that depersonalization is not a neurosis or a psychosis, but a quantitative disturbance in the cathexis of the ego feeling and the ego boundary.

This elucidation of the depersonalized state leads us to an important difference from the out-of-body state—in depersonalization, the shift of the cathexis from the bodily ego to a secondary reinvestment in the body scheme does not occur as it does in OBE. The absence of this bouyant sense of wholeness accompanying the bodily ego feeling contributes to the sensation that depersonalization is dreamlike, unpleasant, and strange. Federn describes this depersonalized feeling as "ego atony." Hence, persons who have episodes of depersonalization do not ordinarily report the sensation of having a "second body," in contrast to OBE subjects.

As we move further down the continuum of states of altered mind/body perception toward the more pathological end, we encounter schizophrenic boundary disturbances. In depersonalization, although the ego has lost its inner coherent unity, no false reality is yet attributed to thought, as in schizophrenia. The loss of ego cathexis in depersonalization differs from that of schizophrenia in that it is much more specific. Federn notes that only the libido component of the ego cathexis is withdrawn in depersonalization. Schizophrenia is characterized by a devastating loss of cathexis of both mental and bodily ego boundaries. A massive confusion of what is inside and what is outside, that is, what is mental content and what is external reality, results from this loss of ego boundaries. Reality testing is sacrificed, and mental contents seem real since the normally functioning ego boundaries have disappeared and no longer differentiate inner from outer. In addition, with this catastrophic collapse of ego boundaries, the schizophrenic patient cannot differentiate himself or herself from persons in the environment and begins to experience fusion with other figures. The OBE subject with intact ego boundaries has no problem differentiating himself or herself from objects in the environment, nor does the individual who suffers depersonalization, even though his or her ego boundaries have been impaired to a certain extent. Hence, at this end of the continuum, there is dissociation between the bodily ego and the mental ego as is present at the other end of the continuum (OBE). However, in addition to that disruption, there is profound impairment in ego feeling and in ego and body boundaries, unlike the situation of the prototypical OBE subject.

This discussion of schizophrenia provides a forum to discuss the problem of reality testing in general in various forms of altered mind/body perception. As we noted in Chapter Six, 94 percent of our OBE subjects firmly believe that their experience was "more real than a dream." How were they aware that this experience was "real" as opposed to "hallucinatory"? Federn points out that the perception of something as real depends not simply on the stimuli entering the physical sense organs but also on the fact that they enter the external dynamic ego boundary, which, of course, includes the sense organs. An object in the environment is sensed as real, without the assistance of any reality testing whatsoever, when its impressions impinge upon a well-cathected ego boundary. This boundary differentiates what is "inner" from what is "outer." When a mental element is included within the ego boundary, which is experienced as ego feeling, the element is mental, that is, it is perceived as a thought. On the other hand, when the element is outside the mental and the bodily ego, that is, not included within the ego cathexis, the element is viewed as a real object.

Turning to the out-of-body experience, as we noted previously, a full ego feeling and an intact ego boundary are both present in the out-of-body state. Therefore, percepts experienced in that state are viewed as real because they impinge on an intact ego boundary. Whether or not they contradict reality as we know it, they are nevertheless perceived as real because of the operation of the ego boundary, just as a dream image may strike us as real despite its contradicting reality. When the external ego boundary loses its cathexis, as in depersonalization, external objects, however distinctly they may be perceived, are sensed as strange, unfamiliar, or even unreal. This mechanism underlies derealization and depersonalization. In the schizophrenic patient loss of reality consists of losing both mental and bodily ego boundary cathexes. Ordinarily, whatever is sensed as mere thought is a mental process that lies inside these boundaries, while whatever is sensed as being real lies outside the boundaries. With no ego boundary whatsoever, there is no means of differentiating what is real from what is thought, which is one of the central features of the schizophrenic process. Federn argues this point of view by pointing out the similarity between hypnagogic ideation and schizophrenic ideation. He notes that the hypnagogic change at the brink of sleep consists of the fading away of the ego and the ego boundary. In a similar fashion the ego boundary disappears in schizophrenia and produces the perceptual hallucinatory experiences, which the schizophrenic cannot differentiate from reality.

The continuum outlined previously is merely a skeletal framework within which we can begin to understand these phenomena using existing knowledge of general psychoanalytic principles of mental functioning. The continuum is not comprehensive and all inclusive. The near-death experience, for example, is not included, although it has many elements similar to those of the out-of-body experience. However, it also has its own unique features that complicate the picture, such as loss of consciousness, compromised physiological states, and the more apparent defensive function. Psychedelic experiences on hallucinogenic drugs might also be included on the lower end of the continuum near the schizophrenic experiences of bodily distortion, although they have certain characteristics that may discriminate them from the schizophrenic's experience. Just as this continuum is not entirely comprehensive, neither is it completely explanatory of every element of the out-of-body experience. It does not address the accuracy or the mechanism of the subject's sensory perceptions in the out-of-body state. These topics will be taken up in Chapter Thirteen.

Eleven — PROBLEMS OF CAUSATION AND MEANING IN THE OUT-OF-BODY EXPERIENCE

Our excursion into metapsychology in the preceding chapter provided us with a coherent ego psychological framework within which we can understand some of the underlying mechanisms involved in the out-of-body experience. However, many unanswered questions remain. What are the underlying causes of out-of-body experience? What is the meaning of an OBE? How do unconscious factors contribute to the formation and interpretation of an out-of-body experience? To answer questions of this kind, we must turn to in-depth studies of individuals who have reported out-of-body experiences. Such questions cannot be answered with broad, sweeping brush strokes, as each individual's experience has its own fine detailed nuances. The experiences may have as a final common pathway the decathexis of body boundaries and the separation of mental ego cathexis from bodily ego cathexis. Nevertheless, the roads to the final common pathway vary as much as individuals vary. First, however, certain fundamental concepts need to be established.

The notion of psychic determinism is generally considered to be a basic tenet of psychoanalysis. Brenner (1955) defines this concept as follows: "...in the mind as in physical nature about us nothing happens by chance or in a random way. Each psychic event is determined by the ones that preceded it. Events in our mental lives that may seem to be random and unrelated to what went on before are only apparently so. In fact, mental phenomena are no more capable of such a lack of causal connection with what preceded them than are physical ones. Discontinuity in this sense does not exist in mental life" (p. 12). Freud founded psychoanalysis on the bedrock of determinism. One of the core principles he embraced early on in his writings was that of overdetermination, as we noted in Chapter Three in our discussion of depersonalization. Stated simply, this refers to Freud's idea that there is never a single cause for a symptom or a psychological event, but rather a whole set of factors that operate together. Moreover, this specific set of factors are causally sufficient only when acting together. No one factor alone can create the symptom or the event. As Sherwood (1969) has pointed out, the concept of overdetermination is often misused to mean that more than one set of antecedent conditions or causes are alone capable of explaining an effect. Freud was specific in his use of the word to indicate that several factors must operate together to create sufficient cause for the effect. This idea is different than asserting that there are several groups of factors that can produce an event, and each set alone can produce the same result. Nonetheless, Freud also believed the second idea, as Sherwood acknowledges: "Freud clearly held that the causes of behavior were both complex (overdetermined) and multiple (in the sense of there being alternate sets of sufficient conditions)" (p. 181). Hence, we can define two fundamental psychoanalytic concepts for the purposes of our discussion here: 1) *overdetermination*—the notion that any element of intrapsychic life is determined simultaneously by a variety of conscious and unconscious factors, which are causally sufficient only when acting together; and 2) *multiple causation*—the idea that any one causative factor, conscious or unconscious, is good and sufficient for an effect at a given point in time, but at any other point in time or with any other individual, a variety of other single causes may also be good and sufficient.

How then may we apply these concepts to the phenomenon of the out-of-body experience? Our investigation has led us to the firm conclusion that there is no one cause for the experience. It is an oversimplification to assert that one contributing factor is the cause. The search for a single causal explanation is the fundamental fallacy of much of the research in this area, as we discussed in Chapter Seven concerning near-death experiences. The notion of multiple causation is extremely useful in understanding out-of-body experiences. For example, in attempting to apply this concept to the out-of-body experience, it is useful to return to the example of the 29-year-old professor, Dr. P., in the last chapter. The fact that he was fatigued after a long business trip and was looking forward to taking a nap may have been sufficient cause for him to decathect his body boundaries, as a result of his lowered attention cathexis, and to experience himself as "rolling out" of his body. Similarly, the mere quiescence of proprioceptive impulses, as in the case of a meditator, may be sufficient cause at a certain point in time for a certain individual to have an out-of-body experience. That same professor or that same meditator may have an OBE at a later time due to the ingestion of an hallucinogenic drug, may have another on a different occasion after the funeral of his mother due to a wish-fulfilling reunion fantasy where his "soul" would unite with hers, and may on yet another occasion have an OBE following a cardiac arrest. Moreover, any one of these causes might be sufficient in one individual, but not sufficient in another.

Turning now to the concept of overdetermination, we can ascertain that some out-of-body experiences are clearly overdetermined while others may not be. One of the difficulties of this notion is that one is hard pressed to assert definitively that only the collective impact of the several different factors is capable of producing the effect, while any one of them would not. However, it is our clinical experience that the concept accurately reflects the richness and complexity of the human psyche and is a term worth keeping. The manifest content of the dream is a good demonstration of the principle of overdetermination. This content is dependent on such factors as the day residue, somatic stimuli, environmental stimuli, the state of the transference in the analytic situation, the nature of early childhood experiences, and the core developmental conflicts that the dream hopes to resolve. For example a 33-year-old woman in psychoanalysis dreamed that a snake bit her on the leg. This dream content could be facilely dismissed as a fear of phallic penetration, but analysis of the dream revealed it to be the complex, multilayered end product of a variety of factors. In addition to the phallic meaning of the snake, it reflected conflicts around oral aggression and oral sadism stemming from a much earlier psychosexual developmental stage. The choice of the snake was also determined by an early traumatic experience where the woman ingested a poisonous substance, resulting in a nasogastric tube being passed into her stomach (the coiled snake in the dream was symbolic of the coiled nasogastric tube she remembered from the incident). The dreamer's experience on the day prior to the dream also partly determined the choice of the snake in the dream image. She had just seen a horror film where a snake was the instrument of murder.

This discussion of the mechanism of overdetermination in

dreams demonstrates clearly how the border between causes and meaning in intrapsychic events is one that is frequently blurred. Schafer (1978) notes that the concept of overdetermination is increasingly used to refer to meanings rather than causes: "The psychoanalyst refers to the multiple definition of single actions as their overdetermination, even though according to the views now being developed, he or she is referring to meanings rather than causes, and even though it cannot and need not be demonstrated that the analysand has been acting in terms of every one of these meanings, unconsciously or otherwise" (p. 20). Hence, as we delve into our individual case examples, we will be examining unconscious meanings in tandem with unconscious determinants, recognizing that the distinction between the two may be more apparent than real.

The discussion of dreams in this context is appropriate for another reason as well. Dreams are normal mental activities that nevertheless demonstrate mechanisms that may be pathological. Freud certainly recognized this in his magnum opus, the *Interpretation of Dreams*: "Now psychoanalytic research finds no fundamental, but only quantitative, distinctions between normal and neurotic life; and indeed the analysis of dreams, in which repressed complexes are operative alike in the healthy and the sick, shows a complete identity both in their mechanisms and in their symbolisms" (1900, pp. 373-374). Just as we sought to define the metapsychological underpinnings of altered mind/body perception in Chapter Ten according to general psychoanalytic principles of mental functioning, we are similarly concerned here with looking at causation and meaning in the context of both normal and abnormal mental functioning. Indeed, among the five cases that we will present in some depth in this chapter, two are from normal subjects who have not defined themselves as patients nor sought psychiatric treatment. The other three may be viewed as clinical examples. Similarities and differences will be noted as we examine both determinants and meanings.

Our examination of the unconscious factors at work in the out-of-body experience is in no way an attempt to explain all the elements of the experience. We do not endeavor to identify the kind of person who is likely to have an OBE, as our survey failed to delineate any such psychological profile. Nor do we try to account for the paranormal perceptual events reported in connection with out-of-body experience. As we stated at the outset, our primary interest is in the psychology of these experiences. Chapter Thirteen will address some of the parapsychological issues. Prior to examining our individual case examples, a brief review of other psychological theories may be useful.

PSYCHOLOGICAL THEORIES

Depth psychologists, such as psychoanalysts, have written very little on the subject of out-of-body experiences. While the psychoanalytic literature on the doppelgänger phenomenon, autoscopy, and depersonalization is moderate to extensive in quantity, the sources on true OBE are confined to Ehrenwald (1974) and Carl Jung (1963), the latter of whom wrote of his own experience. Ehrenwald relies heavily on the defensive denial of death in his efforts to understand the OBE, as we pointed out in Chapter Seven in our discussion of explanatory hypotheses for near-death experiences. He sees out-of-body experiences as having in common a defensive constellation designed to ward off anxiety originating from the threatened distintegration of the ego, from the breakdown of the body image, and from the fear of death. Although Greyson (1983) and Noyes (1981) comment specifically on near-death experiences rather than on the more general phenomenon of out-of-body experience, they have a psychodynamic view that is similar to Ehrenwald's, in that they understand the out-of-body state as an extension of the defensive detachment seen in depersonalization, where the subject wishes to disavow a connection with the body that is risking annihilation. Greyson further speculates that the report of being "out" of one's body may involve a secondary revision of the actual experience, where the individual attempts to reconstruct and verbalize the experience in a way that is explainable to others.

In Jung's autobiography (1963), he describes in some detail his own out-of-body experience after he fractured his foot. He was floating high above the earth in space. He experienced this state as ecstatic and "utterly real." He understood the experience psychologically as a kind of peak experience in which he had attained an objectivity that is possible only when the self is completely individuated. He felt that he was detached from value judgments and from emotional bonds on earth. Like so many out-of-body experiences, Jung's was an integrating, numinous event that profoundly affected his life and contributed to a belief that there was a realm of existence outside of time and beyond death. Jung's statement about the objectivity achieved in his experience resonates with the finding of our study that OBEs of this kind tend to be associated with psychological health.

While little can be found in the psychoanalytic literature, a number of psychological theories concerning the out-of-body experience have appeared in the parapsychological literature. Rogo (1982) has comprehensively reviewed these psychological models, most of which focus on the paranormal aspects of the experience. Blackmore (1984), rejecting the idea of an actual separation of mind from body, asserts that the out-of-body experience is a combination of imagination and extrasensory perception. She says that the subject's perceptions in the out-of-body state are actually a flawed and inaccurate version of the location in which they find themselves. She explains this viewpoint by postulating a "cognitive map," a memory, albeit a three dimensional one, of the world as we know it, which is activated in the out-of-body experience and mistaken for accurate perception.

Palmer (1978) notes, as we do, that changes in proprioceptive feedback within a subject's body may serve to precipitate the OBE, but he goes on to say that the associated change in the body concept produces anxiety in the individual on an unconscious level, resulting in a threat to the subject's self-concept. This anxiety in turn activates the out-of-body experience as a way of attempting to restore one's individual identity. Ego threat is a central part of Palmer's theory, which allies him with psychoanalytic writers who also view the OBE as defensive in nature. He sees the extrasensory phenomena occurring in conjunction with the OBE as connected to the altered state of consciousness that is conducive to out-of-body experience rather than to the OBE itself. In other words, the altered state of consciousness is primary, while both ESP and OBE are secondary phenomena. Honegger (1979) builds upon Palmer's theory to create her "ego homeostasis" model. She views the OBE as intimately tied to self-esteem regulation. The difference between the subject's intentions or desires and the subject's actual achievements serve as a barometer or homeostatic regulator for the organism in this theory. The out-of-body experience serves a corrective function in this formulation, in that it shores up a deflated ego or humbles an overinflated ego (one suspects that Honegger is really referring to what we now call the self in psychoanalytic theory).

These theories approach the problem from a purely theoretical standpoint and do not derive from detailed psychological case studies. Hence, while the general mechanisms they propose may be of some use in understanding the out-of-body experience, they do not provide a model for understanding the singular and idiosyncratic nature of a given individual's experience, either from the standpoint of causation or from the point of view of the significance of the event to the individual. We will endeavor to fill that void with the following case examples.

CASE 1

Robert Monroe is a businessman from Virginia, now in his sixties, who is one of the most widely known gifted subjects in the OBE literature. He has written a book cataloguing his out-of-body exploits (Monroe 1977) and has founded a private institution devoted to the study of such phenomena—the Monroe Institute of Applied Sciences in Faber, Virginia. He voluntarily submitted himself to indepth psychiatric and psychological evaluation several years prior to the publication of this book. He underwent intensive psychiatric interviewing and a battery of different psychological tests. Psychophysiological studies were also performed, which will be discussed in Chapter Twelve. Monroe has never had psychiatric treatment in any form. He has performed at a high level of functioning throughout his career as producer, businessman, and entrepreneur.

As we delve into his background, we find that he did not have out-of-body experiences until the age of 42. He had an orthodox Southern upbringing with high achieving and successful parents. From an early age Monroe had a fascination with flying. He built model planes as a little boy and learned to fly airplanes when he was only in high school. Later, he became an accomplished glider pilot. He was also preoccupied with the thrill of movement and has wonderful memories of riding on trains. Tolpin (1974) has related such intense interest in flying to a developmental viscissitude of the grandiose fantasy that she calls "The Daedalus Experience." She takes this name, of course, from the myth of Daedalus and Icarus, who longed to fly over the sea and created wax wings for themselves to accomplish this task. Icarus, the son of Daedalus, became intoxicated with his ability to fly and flew too near the sun. The sun melted the wax on his wings, and he plunged into the sea as his father, Daedalus, continued on his way. Tolpin postulates that this myth and the fascination with flying is intimately connected with a certain developmental period where the infant experiences an ecstatic primal pleasure at being flung about by his mother and father and doting relatives. This archaic grandiose fantasy of defying gravity and flying through the air is normally tamed in the process of maturity and channeled into high achievement and other kinds of sublimatory activities. Tolstoy, for example, leapt out of a window at the age of nine in an attempt to fly and suffered a concussion. However, he almost never relinquished the literal belief that he could fly. He had ecstatic notions about merging with the moon, which Tolpin relates to the fantasy of mystical merger with his mother, whom he lost at the age of two. This early grandiose notion was, of course, channeled into extraordinary mastery and creativity in the area of writing. Winston Churchill had a similar background, and at 18 jumped off a bridge onto tree tops. This early grandiosity was gradually transformed from the realm of action into the realm of thought, as in his stirring speeches, such as, "We shall never surrender." Tolpin provides another example of a six-year-old child who leapt off of a merry-go-round in an effort to fly and became furious with his mother because he could not. This wish to fly was later transformed into a wish to fly an airplane.

The fascination with out-of-body "travel" seen in Monroe is likely an adult derivative of this Daedalus fantasy. His childhood grandiose wish is transformed not only into out-of-body experiences as an adult, but also into the creation of an institute devoted to the study of these and other esoteric experiences. Hence, in Monroe we see perhaps a more direct translation of the childhood wish to fly into an adult form of the grandiose wish. However, he has used this interest adaptively and productively rather than in a self-destructive or counterproductive way. It may be that this persistent grandiose wish to fly is more likely to be operative as a determinant in those subjects who have the esoteric variety of out-of-body experience, that is, travels to distant locations and through other realms that are fantastic and inexplicable. This determinant may not apply to the more mundane experiences where one simply finds oneself floating on the ceiling above one's body.

If one of the determinants of Monroe's out-of-body experience is this persistent wish to escape the shackles of the earthbound physical form, what are some of the others? His history indicates that he was free from childhood trauma, and in fact, somewhat indulged with creature comforts. His mother, a dynamic and successful physician, had a certain outlook on life that tended to avoid ugliness and unpleasantness. This attribute also emerges in an analysis of Monroe's personality. Both Monroe and his mother used the defenses of denial and avoidance to a significant extent. These hypomanic defenses against aggression, tragedy, and destructiveness were further demonstrated in projective psychological testing. The Rorschach test indicated that Monroe is a man who avoids many aspects of his internal life. He has strong defenses against dealing with sexuality, defensive feelings, and especially aggression, all areas of his psyche that he prefers to keep out of his awareness. He has a pervasive tendency to avoid and detach himself from feelings, which shows itself in his patterns of thinking, his use of language, and his interpersonal relations. He often simply steers off, away, and tangentially to the way others think, feel, perceive, and express themselves. These personality inclinations contribute to the content of what he saw on a particular inkblot, which is often seen as a bat or a bird. Monroe saw this is "a flying unit, with wings, in the shape of a bird or the body of a butterfly or insect, flying upwards toward the top of the card." Thus, the out-of-body experience in Monroe also serves the function of avoidance of conflict. By transcending the prison of his body, it allows him to steer clear of such potential conflict areas as sexuality, depression, and aggression.

Further testing of Monroe, using the Dickstein Death Anxiety Scale indicated that Monroe's fear of death is actually very low compared with the normal population. Hence, while denial of death may be operative in some subjects, it does not seem to be a central feature in Monroe's out-of-body experiences.

Finally, one other finding worth mentioning is his tendency to keep opposite and contradictory constructs separate from each other and to utilize the energy of the tension between these split-off opposites for creative endeavors. This tendency to maintain contradictory thoughts, feelings, and attitudes in conscious awareness without provoking a great deal of anxiety is often found in creative people. Hence, the experiences of "leaving the body" do not overwhelm and disorganize Monroe since there is little cognitive dissonance ordinarily created by an intense experience that does not fit into the paradigm of Western science. He was able to maintain this experience side-by-side with his rational empirical attitudes about what was necessary for the day-to-day demands of the business world.

CASE 2

Our second subject, like Monroe, is a normal individual who has never been identified as a psychiatric patient or undergone treatment for psychological problems. She also agreed to intensive psychological study. This 35-year-old mother of three children, whom we referred to as Mrs. K. in Chapter Six, has had out-of-body experiences since the age of ten. Three rather vivid out-of-body experiences occurred following her younger sister's death, and one vivid experience took place following the death of her son. If we look into the background of Mrs. K., we find that she was raised by a rigid, harsh father and a loving, supportive mother. The household was often filled with tension because of the conflict between her parents, who finally divorced during her senior year in high school. She described a family in which she was constantly running from and denying the strengths and powers of male figures. She negotiated adolescence without major problems, but she feels that her strict religious practices during that time were enormously helpful to her. Out-of-body experiences during latency and adolescence served as an escape from the turmoil in the household. These liberating experiences were very meaningful to her, even though they were at times frightening in the beginning.

After she married her high school sweetheart and settled down to have a family of three children, one son died. Further out-of-body experiences occurred at this time and became very special and unique. She began to actively seek them. In her own words, "My life and attitude toward OBEs began to really turn around. They sustained me through some very trying times and gave me hope that I don't think there would have been otherwise. They have been invaluable to me and rather than robbing me of my sanity, have succeeded in strengthening it." These experiences at this point in her life probably had the special meaning of a reunion fantasy with her dead son. If she could transcend the limits of her body, perhaps a soul separate from the physical body survives death. This meaning of the OBE filled her with hope about meeting her son again in the "Hereafter."

Another important feature of the above quotation is Mrs. K.'s report that the OBE was an ego-strengthening and integrating experience for her rather than a disorganizing one. Elsewhere (Twemlow et al. 1982), we have proposed that certain kinds of psychic experiences may serve an ego-integrating function. So it is in the case of Mrs. K. and her out-of-body experiences. These served as a denial of death and a denial of mourning, but also provided her with strength to go on in her daily functioning. After her younger sister's death, she had a similar resurgence in frequency and vividness of her out-of-body experiences, confirming this determinant.

Mrs. K. had a very high score on Tellegen's "Absorption" Scale, indicating an exaggerated tendency to focus on internal fantasy. She seems to be a person who can easily become absorbed in her own internal processes. The fact that Mrs. K.'s OBEs were intimately connected with the denial of death, while Monroe's are apparently not underscores the futility and absurdity of searching for one single cause and one single meaning of these experiences. Two normal subjects have phenomenologically similar experiences, but each has his or her own set of causes, meanings, and functions.

To summarize the findings in Mrs. K. and to demonstrate the principles of multiple causation and overdetermination in these experiences, we will now review the principle determinants of her experience: 1) in childhood, the OBE served the function of escape from family tension; 2) following the deaths of her sister and her son, the OBEs served to deny the reality of death and the decomposition of the body by confirming to her that a soul apart from the physical body survived death; 3) during the period of mourning after the death of her relatives, the OBE instilled a sense of hope in her—hope that a reunion with her loved ones was possible in a realm beyond earthly existence; 4) the OBEs in Mrs. K. served an ego-integrating function in times of crisis, which helped her master conflict and inner turmoil through an ecstatic transcendence of the body; and 5) her tendency to attune herself to internal states seemed to facilitate the vivid imagery she described in her out-of-body experiences.

It seems that Mrs. K.'s out-of-body experiences had different functions at different points in her life. She was able to use her experiences adaptively like Monroe, to sustain her sense of psychic equilibrium and to provide herself with a sense of meaning and purpose.

CASE 3

While Case 1 and 2 are normal subjects, we also wish to demonstrate in this chapter how the out-of-body experience may interface with psychopathological issues at various levels of severity in the spectrum of psychiatric disorders. We shall first examine the case of a neurotic man who came to psychoanalysis. It is perhaps worth mentioning that, to our knowledge, this example is the first case report in the literature of a neurotic subject with out-of-body experiences who has come under psychoanalytic scrutiny. Mr. Q., as we shall call this subject, was a 37-year-old professional man, who came to analysis with a variety of neurotic inhibitions around sexuality and aggression that presented obstacles to his success in the professional arena and in the realm of interpersonal relationships. He had had two out-of-body experiences as an adult, both of the mundane variety and had developed an active interest in the out-of-body phenomenom. In fact he sought one of us out for treatment because he was aware of our research in this area.

Early in the treatment of Mr. Q., it became apparent that his attitude toward his body was characterized by loathing, disgust, and repulsion. Raised as a strict Roman Catholic, he remembered sitting in church many a Sunday and staring at a stained glass window depicting the Ascension of Christ. This notion of the potential of transcending one's physical body had enormous appeal to Mr. Q. He would avoid touching his genitals as a teenager, let alone masturbate, and was extremely inhibited about the prospect of sexual relations. He seriously considered the priesthood as a profession. He recalled that the asceticism and self-denial of the life of a monk were very attractive to him. He was a perfectionist who saw analysis as an opportunity to become "even more perfect." He believed very strongly that his pursuit of perfection would result in immortality, the ultimate perfect state. He dreaded the possibility of the extinction of his consciousness at death and longed to believe that if he did everything properly, his consciousness would survive in a heavenly existence. He was consumed with thoughts of purifying himself of all bodily needs and urges. He had intense shame over his bodily functions and had embarassing dreams of defecating in his pants in public. He used excessive amounts of toilet paper to eradicate any trace of feces. As he went back further in his childhood in the course of analysis, he recalled hearing his parents making grunting and groaning noises through the walls of his bedroom at night. He tried to understand these noises as something other than what they were—the sounds of sexual intercourse. He denied that his parents ever had intercourse and became extremely angry at a chum of his who told him, when he was ten years old, that his parents had to have had intercourse to conceive him. He adamantly denied that his parents had ever had intercourse and asserted that he had come into the world by some other means. His father had been gone for long periods of time during his latency years, and the patient was quite threatened by the availability of his mother. Hence, his body also began to carry the meaning of a potential instrument of incestuous gratification.

The out-of-body experience in this individual then had a variety of meanings. It served as a vehicle for the ultimate transcendence into a perfect state free from bodily needs and desires, particularly forbidden incestuous desires for his mother, who was far too available to him. It meant a merger with Christ in a blissful, beatific union. A horrible existential dread lay at the core of this patient, and the out-of-body experience represented to him a triumph over the terror that his body would ultimately decay and his consciousness would be extinguished. Ernest Becker's comments on this existential problem are pertinent in this context: "The body is definitely the hurdle for man, the decaying drag of the species on the inner freedom and purity of his self. The basic problem of life, in this sense, is whether the species, the body, will predominate over one's individuality (inner self)...the emotional message is that they have no control over their fate or that the accidentality of the body form inhibits and restricts freedom and determines them" (1973, p. 226). Becker also notes how anal concerns are intimately linked to existential anxiety as well as to the classical Freudian issues of autonomy and control related to psychosexual development. He observes that all of man's pretenses of transcendence and defiance of the body are shattered by the fact of decay represented by defecation: "Anxiety over the body shows up, too, in all 'anal' dreams, when people find themselves soiled by overflowing toilets, someone spashing urine—in the midst of the most important affairs and all dressed up in their social finery. No mistake—the turd is mankind's real threat. We see this confusion between symbolic transcendence and anal function throughout the psychoanalytic literature" (p. 227, 1973). Hence, in Mr. Q., the OBE had the meaning of a pathway by which he could escape the reminders of his own mortality and his own decaying and dying body.

A final consideration in the case of Mr. Q. was the transference meaning of his out-of-body experiences. He sought out an analyst with an interest in out-of-body experiences and imagined that he would be the most interesting patient in his analyst's case load. He knew that he and his analyst shared a special interest, and he believed that there was a special bond between them as a result of this shared interest. The patient often denied the existence of the analyst's other patients and thought of himself as a special only child. This transference development was related to intense sibling rivalry with his brothers and sisters during his childhood, particularly for his father's attention. When he actually had an out-of-body experience one evening, he came to analysis the next day with extraordinary enthusiasm. He said he could not wait to tell his analyst, knowing that his analyst would love to hear about the experience.

The case of Mr. Q. demonstrates nicely how the out-of-body experience can be overdetermined. A variety of needs, wishes, defenses, and conflicts coalesce around one intrapsychic event. Of particular interest in this case is the determinant involving the wish to escape the body because of its association with incestuous wishes and gratification. This same determinant was involved in Miss D. and Mrs. F., two of the cases of depersonalization described in Chapter Three. Comparing the case of Mr. Q. with these two cases of depersonalization demonstrates how similar determinants may result in different intrapsychic experiences, depending on the ego strengths of the individual and his or her ability to use the experience adaptively rather than to succumb to the experience and react in an anxious, disorganized manner. To use an analogy from genetics, the experiences may have genotypic similarities, but their phenotypic expressions are different.

The comparison of the case of Mr. Q. with the two cases of depersonalization also serves to demonstrate the similarities and differences of the defensive functions of the out-of-body experience and of depersonalization. While there are many individual defense mechanisms, the psychoanalytic concept of defense, as a general notion, refers to the manner in which the psyche protects itself from being overwhelmed by various affects and impulses. At first blush it might seem that depersonalization is clearly defensive, in that it often occurs in response to a precipitating stress, while OBE is less clearly defensive, given the fact that it usually occurs in a calm, relaxed state. However, our examination of the normal research subjects, as well as the analytic data from Mr. Q., indicates that a variety of defensive functions can also be attributed to out-of-body experiences. The primary difference seems to be that depersonalization can be characterized as a response to a more obvious and more immediate threat or stress, for example, an automobile accident or performance in front of a live audience, whereas the nature of the threat in OBE is less immediate, more obscure, and more intrapsychic than external. In the two cases of depersonalization as a defense against anxiety about the body as an instrument of incestuous gratification, one of the patients (Miss D.) was responding to a real external threat from her stepfather, while the other's depersonalization occurred in the context of a psychotic decompensation with delusions about such a threat (Mrs. F.). In contrast Mr. Q.'s concerns stemmed only from childhood fantasy, not from reality, and were largely repressed until the process of analysis brought them to the surface.

The ego in depersonalization is more apt to be overwhelmed because of the greater intensity of the threat as compared to out-of-body experience, where the full, intact ego feeling is preserved. Similarly, in depersonalization the experience is assimilated by the ego as a pathological and distressing experience that requires psychiatric attention, while the OBE tends to be assimilated by the ego as an exhilarating, mind-expanding, and integrating experience. Hence, one can conclude that it is the ego's response to the experience that differentiates the out-of-body experience from depersonalization, rather than the presence or absence of defensive functions in the experience.

CASE FOUR

Ms. R. was a 38-year-old secretary who volunteered herself for intensive study as part of our research. She had been married four times and was living alone at the time of the evaluation. She reported that her experiences began as flying dreams in childhood. Her first true out-of-body experience occurred in the third grade after she was humiliated and scolded in class. Noteworthy past history in Ms. R. included the fact that her mother had died of polio when Ms. R. was only six. Most of her out-of-body experiences had occurred when she was in her twenties and early thirties. In her mid-twenties she was studying mysticism and began to try to leave her body through conscious efforts. She would lie in bed and withdraw all sensation from her limbs, trunk, and chest. Her extremities would get cold. She said that spirits invaded and shook the body while she was out. "Negative entities" sniffed around the body and tried to take it over, according to Ms. R. In contrast to these unpleasant and revolting beings, was a man named Duke who accompanied her in her out-of-body experience. She reported that he reached out to her and lifted her out of her body. He took her over a beautiful, clear ocean and communicated with her in such a way that she understood things like she never had understood them before. She described the experience as "incredibly real" and definitely different from a dream. The man who accompanied her explained to her that she was one of a special group that they had taken to study. After returning to her body, she would question all of her values. She had a tremendous sense of power and energy and did not know what she could do with it.

Intensive psychiatric interviewing and projective psychological testing indicated that Ms. R. was diagnosable as a borderline personality disorder. Indeed, she had been involved in psychotherapy several times for brief periods throughout her adult life. She had never required hospitalization. Her reality testing was generally intact, as is typical of borderline patients, except around two major problem areas: management of affect and object relations. Regarding affect, her Rorschach responses indicated that she attempts to stay away from feelings and in the process, utilizes a variety of defenses including isolation of affect, denial, and suppression. If these defenses falter, as they tend to do when confronted with affect of an intense nature, whether it be painful, angry, fearful, or sad, Ms. R.'s reality testing begins to deteriorate, and she tends to decompensate in a paranoid direction.

In the other principal problem area, we found that Ms. R.'s relations with others are highly colored by remnants of an intensely symbiotic, hostile-dependent relationship with her mother. Separation-individuation was found to be the primary developmental task for this woman. Her approach to the world and to those around her was typical of young children with school phobia, that is, the world is experienced as a hostile, frightening place outside the mutually protective mother-child embrace. Ms. R. tends to deal with this projected threat by minimizing and denying it, but when the fear of separation become sufficiently intense, psychological disruption ensues. Males and male sexuality are a source of considerable anxiety for Ms. R., as it is seen as part of the hostile external world outside of the mother-infant dyad. She saw men as only interested in sex, wanting their "pound of flesh." She said that she had come to a point in her life where she could have more personal growth without men: "If you have a man, he sucks your energy. He always bleeds things off you." She reported that she had noted that she had more energy for things like out-of-body experience when she remained celibate. Men were perceived as a "negative draw" on her energy. She described her last husband as like a "black widow spider, who sucked me dry as a shell like a cicada." She kept away from him because he seemed to sap all her energy from her. She even avoided being touched by men because of this concern that they would suck energy away from her.

From our careful study of Ms. R., we were able to trace several determinants of her out-of-body experiences. For Ms. R., the OBE was clearly a means of release from intensely painful feelings. This function of the OBE was seen in her response to Card IX of the Rorschach: "A person walking into a hazy area, walking from something definite and harsh, passing through a happy area, and on the other side, it's much more calm, there is light reflected on the portion of the gate that is open, but I can't see anything beyond the gate." The similarity to some of the imagery in the near-death experience is clear in this response. Hence, the OBE is a passage from the painful, harsh land of unpleasant feelings into a calm, tranquil paradise. Again, as with Mrs. M., we see the ego-integrating function of the OBE. Since projective testing indicated that the patient is likely to psychotically decompensate under the pressure of intense affect, the out-of-body experience, as a release from these affects, is a much more adaptive way of coping with these overwhelming emotions.

Separation anxiety seemed to be the core anxiety in Ms. R., as is the case with most borderline patients. It is interesting to note in this regard that she saved the sloughed-off remnant of the umbilical cord of her son for many years. Separation anxiety is another source of psychological disruption, as mentioned previously, and another function of her out-of-body experiences was an attempt to master separation. She would counterphobically leave her body in this effort at mastery, but was accompanied by the idealized male guide. The ultimate separation, of course, is death, and her out-of-body experiences can be viewed as a trial run for death as the ultimate and final separation. The similarities of the Card IX response to the near-death experience lend further credence to this idea. Moreover, the assistance of her guide, Duke, reassures her that separation is nothing to be feared as one will not actually be alone. Closely related to this concern about separation is a rebirth theme. It was amazing how frequently Ms. R. made reference to cicadas in the course of her evaluation. On Card I of the Rorschach, she saw a "cicada with a chunky body and wings." She elaborated further on this image: "Cicadas amaze me; imagine the trauma they go through getting out with their wings; it must be a great relief when they get out, but it must be difficult getting out. I've never seen it happen. I wonder if that is what is happening while all that screeching is going on in the spring." The separation experience from the shedded body of the cicada is like a birth experience, painful but necessary. Her out-of-body experiences have the psychological meaning of giving birth to a new self, who is no longer hindered by the shedded body.

Finally, the OBE as described with her male guide, Duke, can be viewed as a "cleaned up" sexual experience. Sexuality was a major conflict area for Ms. R., and was seen as something "bad," where men sapped her energy and extracted their "pound of flesh." Having shed this impure body and set off on a flight above the ocean with Duke, she was capable of an exhilarating experience with a man free from the ugliness she associated with her body. As long ago as 1900, Freud linked flying dreams with sexual experiences. The men in these experiences are split into good objects (Duke) and bad objects, who sniff around the shedded body while she is out of it. This characteristic splitting of objects in her environment into good and bad is typical of borderline object relations.

Overdetermination is again clearly applicable to the experiences of Ms. R. Although she was more severely disturbed than the neurotic Mr. Q., she is still capable of functioning at a nonpsychotic level in her work and in superficial relationships. As with Mrs. K., her OBEs may actually help her maintain some degree of psychological intactness. Her ego strength is still sufficiently adequate to allow her to integrate the experience and use it adaptively. The same cannot be said of those individuals at the lower end of the psychopathological spectrum, as our next case illustrates.

CASE 5

As we noted in the preceding chapter, the diagnosis of schizophrenia in no way precludes the possibility that an out-of-body experience might occur. An OBE in a schizophrenic patient would most likely not have phenomenological features identical to those of the prototypical OBE because that experience presumes a certain amount of ego integration and intact reality testing. However, a modified version of the OBE can indeed occur, as the following brief example illustrates. Mr. S. was a 21-year-old schizophrenic young man in an inpatient unit of a psychiatric hospital. He woke up in the middle of the night and described the following experience: "I got out of bed and sat down on the floor next to the bed. I must have gone into an astral projection since my body stayed in the bed. I saw my brother lying in the bed, looking dead. His spirit was trapped in my body. I felt like I was floating up in the room. I was scared, looking at my brother in my body. When the staff entered the room, I went back into my body."

In terms of causation, we can understand that upon waking up, Mr. S.'s body boundaries, ordinarily weakly cathected due to his schizophrenic illness, may have had even more cathexis withdrawn from them because of the patient's attentional state. When he experienced himself as disconnected from the body, he reacted differently from the prototypical OBE subject who does not suffer from schizophrenia. He delusionally elaborated the experience by deciding that his physical body must be possessed by his brother, who in turn, must be dead. The only way his brother's spirit could be trapped in his body would be for the brother to be dead. This delusional elaboration undoubtedly activated anxieties about his death wish toward his brother. Hence, instead of reacting in the pleasant or ecstatic way that the normal subject reacts, he became terrified during the experience. This short vignette indicates how the meaning of the OBE can be vastly different to an individual who lacks the ego capacity to integrate the experience and put it in a context that is understandable and acceptable.

The schizophrenic patient is chronically burdened with the problems of integrating his mind with his body. Whereas the normal or prototypical OBE subject has a secure mind-body relationship ordinarily and can accept such extraordinary states of consciousness within that framework, the schizophrenic has no such comfort. He has never had a secure seating in his body and relies instead on a hypermagnification of mental processes.

The principle of overdetermination is also a principle of multiple function (Waelder 1930). We hope that in providing these detailed analyses of case examples, we have demonstrated that the out-of-body experience has a variety of functions within the human psyche. These functions vary across individuals and in the same individual across time. Moreover, we hope that we have raised serious questions about oversimplified, unicausal theories of OBE that link all experiences to one underlying issue. The principles of multiple causation and overdetermination seem to be the most useful concepts in elucidating the problems of causation and meaning in the out-of-body experience.

Twelve — PSYCHOPHYSIOLOGICAL CORRELATES OF THE OUT-OF-BODY EXPERIENCE

The problem of knowing what is "really real" is an ongoing theme throughout this book. Those oriented toward neurophysiology treat data derived by laboratory instrumentation as more real and more reliable than the more mentalistic "subjective" data. However, modern holographic theories of mind (Bohm 1980; Comfort 1981), beyond the scope of this book, indicate that there is no reason to suppose that physical matter has any more "realness" than "mental matter." Neurobiology is as complex and as flexible as the mental phenomena that comprise thinking. For example a recent editorial in *Trends in Neuro Science* (*Brain/Mind Bulletin*, 1983) noted: "The flow of information through neural circuits is more dynamic than previously imagined." It appears that, for example, the brain is quite capable of adapting to instantaneous changes in input by making use of regulator genes that quickly change their function as required. A neurobiologist, Rose (1980), after 20 years of work in the field, says that we "have to abandon the concept of cause as inappropriate and confusing." He goes on to say, "specific biochemical states correspond to specific behavioral states, not because of a chemistry that causes the behavior, but because it is the behavior at a different level of analysis expressed in a different language."

For the sake of completeness, we will review in this chapter, the few available studies of the electrophysiological correlates of the out-of-body experience and report our own findings in two cases of

---

*This chapter was coauthored by Mr. Paul Shannon of Afton, Virginia.

out-of-body experience, one in an experimental subject who was naive to the purpose of the experiment and the other in an adept subject. We will then suggest possible interpretations of those data.

One of the difficulties in understanding the out-of-body experience is that the experience can occur in a variety of different states, varying from coma through normal alertness. People adept at producing out-of-body experiences quite frequently produce the experiences while in a normal waking state and without any unusual induction ritual (Osis et al. 1977). Besides states of physical and mental relaxation, out-of-body experiences with near-death features occur in states associated with pain and in a variety of other highly traumatic situations (see Chapters Seven, Eight, and Nine).

LABORATORY INVESTIGATIONS

Psychophysiological data on the out-of-body experience are variable in quality. This observation is not surprising in view of the fact that there is no reliable way of inducing an OBE and no definite agreement on the descriptive characteristics of the experience. In a weakly supported piece of speculative research, Salley (1982) suggests that out-of-body experiences might occur "in the context of the physiology of REM sleep; but in a state of clear wakeful-like consciousness" (p. 162). He uses anecdotal material such as reported penile erection in the case of Robert Monroe to suggest that dream-like REM states might be occurring. Rogo (1984), representing the unambivalent dualist, states that if some substance is really leaving the body during the OBE, it is logical to assume that some form of neurophysiological alteration would accompany its departure. Thus, he is looking for further validation of the "reality" of mind-body separation, a point to which we will return in Chapter Thirteen.

Tart (1967, 1968) reports studies of two subjects. One woman was a personal friend of Tart's, and as he points out, "One can never describe one's friends objectively." A periodic, severe psychiatric illness in this woman required Stelazine, which can cause slow waves on the EEG tracing, hence confounding the picture, although Tart felt she was probably not on Stelazine at the time of the experiment. All of her frequent experiences occurred during sleep and were descriptively typical of the mundane type OBE (Chapter One). She found herself floating near the ceiling, apparently wide awake, and observed her physical body lying on the bed. These OBEs had occurred since childhood, and she had learned to accept them as ordinary. She was monitored in a sleep laboratory over a two month period. She had a great deal of REM activity early in stage 1 sleep, which is unusual. She also had vivid hypnagogic imagery. Three out-of-body experiences occurred in a total of four nights in the laboratory. Tart reports that, "It is difficult to state conclusively what type of EEG pattern accompanied floating experiences, and the full out-of-body experience, since it was difficult to locate when these experiences had occurred, 'retrospectively'" (p. 19). Tart feels that the experiences occurred during a poorly developed Stage 1 alpha pattern that was dominated by alphoid activity mixed with transitory periods of wakefulness (alphoid activity includes alpha mixed with sleep spindles). This alphoid activity was always 1–1½ cycles per second slower than her normal alpha rhythm, and was not accompanied by rapid eye movements, alterations in skin resistance, or change in heart rate. Many ordinary REM sleep periods without out-of-body experiences were recorded in the laboratory. In a second study (reported first in 1967), a male subject, Mr. X, was monitored for nine sessions over a period of approximately nine months. Mr. X., in fact, later turned out to be Robert Monroe. Although he is treated anonymously in Tart's paper, he subsequently became well-known for the publication of his book, *Journeys Out of the Body*. He did not object to the revelation that he was the subject of this experiment. We were subsequently also able to perform some psychophysiological experiments on Monroe in our own laboratory in 1976, the results of which are reported later in this chapter.

While monitoring Monroe's EEG, electroculogram (EOG), and heart rate, Tart concluded that, as with Mrs. Z., Monroe has his out-of-body experiences in "borderline" states, that is, the state between sleep and wakefulness dominated by alphoid rhythms. Some of his brief out-of-body experiences occurred during REM sleep, what Tart called State 1 REM periods. Actually, the only similarity between Tart's two subjects was that both were somewhere between sleeping and wakefulness and both had mixed EEGs, with some characteristics similar to relaxed light sleep and others similar to features of an alert and aroused state.

Many adept subjects are able to produce their out-of-body experiences while awake, even while quite alert. EEG data from Blue Harary (Morris et al. 1978; Hartwell et al. 1975) were taken over 13 sessions. Sophisticated multivariate analyses were applied to the data, and each analysis showed that the OBE state, as reported by Blue

Harary, differed from the non-OBE state in three of the variables measured: 1) respiration rate showed a statistically significant increase while in the out-of-body-state; 2) heart rate showed a similar change; while, 3) skin potential decreased significantly, also indicating a high arousal state. EEG data were analyzed for both alpha density and frequency in each cerebral hemisphere, but no significant differences were found. Neither did the eye movement or electromyogram (EMG) data show significant differences. The EEG tracings during the out-of-body experience were read as "normal, waking, eyes closed," by an experienced clinical electroencephalgrapher. As a matter of fact, in the case of Harary, contrary to Salley's view, eye movements actually decreased during the out-of-body states. The investigators felt that neither the absent eye movements nor the high alpha content of the EEG were compatible with light sleep or with REM dreams. The subject appeared to be in a "deeply relaxed, but waking" state.

Palmer (1979) studied extrasensory perception and its correlation with out-of-body experiences. Analysis of parietal EEG power in the beta, alpha, theta and delta bands demonstrated that when in an out-of-body state, three out of 20 subjects showed more than "30 percent theta in their baseline EEG's." These three subjects all reported more vivid OBEs than the remaining 17 subjects.

A study of a well known psychic and artist, Mr. Ingo Swann, is reported by Osis (1977). This particular experiment studied 45 instances of his OBEs. A relatively unsophisticated EEG analysis was used. The EEG's were hand scored with analysis of alpha, beta, and theta patterns, using a digital frequency discriminator. Osis concludes that, "Regardless of other interventions, such as biofeedback training, with this subject we found a low voltage mixed activity pattern, usually prominent when Ingo reported being out of his body" (p. 531). The subject himself felt that high amplitude alpha and theta may be associated with introspection and with pinpointing details (during an OBE), while a low voltage mixed pattern might be associated with awareness of the whole scene and decision-making abilities involved in perception. This speculation is curious in that it implies that the parapsychological question of whether mind actually separates from body is a rather empty one, since the hypothesized changes in the EEG suggest a rather strong persisting link with the brain substance!

In Swann's case there was a cessation of eye movements when he reported being in the out-of-body state. In fact Swann felt that these movements distracted him from his OBE vision. Hence, he sometimes wore a blindfold to keep his eyes from moving. Breathing and blood volume remained quite normal. Osis also reports that, "the same sort of EEG changes that we have found in association with Ingo's OBE periods were also found when he was asked to do some mental problem-solving, but the amplitude decreases were greater" (p. 533).

One tentative conclusion from these findings is that the subjects themselves enter self-consistent brain states when they report out-of-body experiences. We seriously doubt that the EEG's reported in these four studies, if scored by blind raters, could distinguish the out-of-body state from other mixed states of light sleep and relaxed wakefulness.

THE OBE PSYCHOPHYSIOLOGY OF ROBERT MONROE

Observations of Robert Monroe were made by one of us, (S.W.T.) and a colleague, Dr. Fowler Jones of the University of Kansas Medical Center, over a 30-minute time period when Monroe was monitored by a Beckman polygraph with left and right occipital EEG electrodes. He was observed by us through a one-way window (Twemlow 1977). Most striking was Monroe's spasmodic breathing with periods of apnea. After these apneic periods, the breaths were gulping. Simultaneously, Dr. Jones and S.W.T. turned to each other and reported the impression of a heat-wave-like distortion beginning at Monroe's waist, so that it was difficult to get a clearly focused picture of his upper body, although his lower body was in clear focus. Previously, Monroe had stated that he would be able to get out of his body quickly but could not signal it, although he could signal within five seconds of return. This distortion disappeared rather suddenly a little before he roused himself. At that time his EEG showed a shift in high amplitude patterns to the right hemisphere with a low amplitude in the left occipital lead.

He seemed to wake without anxiety, although he was moderately disoriented in space for about 30 seconds, with slight slurring of his speech. He could not recapture his experience immediately. His galvanic skin resistance (GSR) level during the session showed an increase in arousal of approximately 150 microvolts, marked by the total absence of either specific or nonspecific responses during his out-of-body phase. At one point, when a technician entered the room to check electrodes, Monroe appeared to be unaware of his presence, and there was no fluctuation in GSR. The skin of his arm and forearm were dry and warm to the touch.

Sections of Monroe's EEG during this reported out-of-body experience were analyzed for frequency differences both within and between hemispheres. An analysis of variance was run, with the data divided into beginning, middle, and end sections, each section having 29 values for a total of 290 seconds. Two groups were analyzed: right and left hemispheres. There seemed to be no significant frequency differences between hemispheres, although the amplitude differences were obvious. There were significant differences between the beginning and middle, the middle and end, and the beginning and end sections of Monroe's EEG in each hemisphere. This latter difference ($F=41.47$ and $F=59.08$; $p<.001$) showed that the "before" and "after" OBE frequencies were much higher than the "during" OBE frequencies. Standard deviations were also significantly smaller with the middle section as compared to the beginning and end sections. A power spectral analysis of OBE periods showed power peaks at 4-5 Hertz with very little activity above 10 Hertz.

What are we to conclude from this experiment? Although the observational findings were more provocative than the EEG findings, they are less easily explained. Clearly, Monroe was in a state of deep relaxation. In addition, when in his out-of-body state, there is a frequency slowing, with an interesting shift in power to a 4–5 Hertz range, the theta-delta transitional zone. This electrophysiological borderline state correlates closely with Tart's findings and Harary's reference to borderline sleep-wakefulness states. Its significance is further explicated by the unusual findings in the case of our second subject, Ms. Y., whom we will discuss later in the chapter.

All of these studies indicate that neurophysiological change might well accompany the out-of-body experience, but there is no indication that any stable, directly correlating state exists. Actually, it is not even clear whether the states are the cause or the effect of the out-of-body experience. Although it is certainly possible that different individuals have different OBE brain wave states, one consistent subjective correlate of these psychophysiological studies is that subjects appeared to be between states, that is, in transitional states, either in the frequency domain, in the case of Monroe (between theta and delta), between deep sleep and light sleep, or between light sleep and the hypnagogic state. Sometimes, paradoxical states exist, such as Blue Harary's and Ingo Swann's states of "relaxed wakefulness." Swann had a degree of alertness, sufficient to perform complex cognitive acts, co-existing with a state normally indicative of little cognitive activity, that is, a state of relaxation.

These reports suggest the possibility that the out-of-body experience is a phenomenon occurring during a change of state rather than in one particular stable state. The shifting from one state to another, whether this be from normal to high arousal (NDE), light sleep to deep sleep, or deep sleep to coma, when no stable electrophysiological state exists may be the optimal condition for the out-of-body experience to occur.

THE CASE OF MS. Y.

Ms. Y. was a 23-year-old white female who had had some college education. She was left-handed with mixed dominance. At the time of the experiment she was separated from her husband, a severely disturbed man who physically abused her from time to time. She subsequently divorced him. She worked as a clerk-typist for a large institution and was entirely reliable in her work habits. She had a long-standing interest in psychological phenomena, in general, but no particular focus on mystical pursuits. She volunteered for the experiment in answer to an advertisement. The experiment was designed to assess the sleep-inducing effects of binaural acoustic stimulation using audio tapes. A single-subject, intensive time series design was used where the subject was exposed to conditions of tape on five minutes, tape off five minutes in an A-B-A mode. Periodic sampling of the left and right occipital electroencephalogram was made at intervals during these conditions. Subjects were divided into two groups: 1) those who were given Robert Monroe's book, *Journeys Out-of-the-Body* to read and to whom it was suggested that the experiment would induce out-of-body experiences, and 2) those who were told nothing at all about the purpose of the experiment. The subject, Ms. Y., was in the latter "naive" group. Standard instructions were given that the subjects should relax and listen to the taped sounds through headphones and simply let their thoughts wander.

Four different forms of binaural acoustical tapes were used in twice weekly sessions for a total of eight sessions. Before and after each taped session, self-scored measures of anxiety were made; temperature, barometric pressure, and relative humidity were measured; and the subject was debriefed according to a standardized format. This debriefing was audio-taped and was later transcribed. Ms. Y. was administered the Differential Personality Inventory (Tellegen 1976) and the Imaginal Process Inventory (Singer and Antrobus 1972). Results of the complete study with 11 subjects will be reported elsewhere. Here we will focus exclusively on the case of Ms. Y., who, during the last tape condition, had a fortuitously recorded out-of-body experience.

A Beckman type polygraph was used with regular Beckman electrodes. A 10–20 standard bipolar electrode placement was made. The electrode placement was right occipital (0_2) referenced to the right earlobe (A_2), left occipital (0_1) referenced to the left earlobe (A_1), and a center forehead ground position. Ms. Y. sat in a reclining chair in a dimly lighted room. Visual observations were made through a one-way window. The data were recorded on standard I.R.I.G. 7-channel analog FM tape. Due to the wide-band nature of the Beckman polygraph the data were recorded in the I.R.I.G. 1.25 KHz bandwidth mode. The two data channels were digitized so that 1,024 samples spanned five seconds of collected data. This sample rate was chosen after visually displaying the recorded data to determine the maximum frequency extent in the Fourier domain. The maximum frequencies did not exceed normal beta frequencies, so that after applying the Nyquist criterion, there was a potentially useful bandwidth of 102.4 hertz and a frequency resolution of 0.2 hertz. For display purposes the data were not plotted beyond 20.8 hertz, as no significant activity was detected beyond that frequency. The amplitude time plots are direct plots of the digitized data, which spanned 15-second intervals to characterize adequately the brain activity at the time of recording. In order to characterize qualitative frequencies for the states of consciousness, averages of Fourier samples were also taken over the several-minute data collection periods. Before and after the session, the subject had a very low self-report anxiety level, with little differences between the before and after measures. At the time of the session the laboratory temperature was 70° F, relative humidity 63 percent, barometric pressure 30.63 mm of mercury and rising. These values remained constant during the session.

Psychological test measures delineated a specific personality profile for Ms. Y. On the Differential Personality Inventory she scored in the 40th percentile range for social potency, 12th percentile for impulse control, 14th percentile for danger-seeking versus harm avoidance, and 88th percentile for absorption. Thus, she can be characterized as not socially conscious, quite impulsive, actively danger-seeking, and high on the absorption score. She is more similar to our NDE subjects than to our out-of-body subjects, especially in the absorption score. The Imaginal Process Inventory is a 400-item measure with 20 subscales having to do specifically with either content or structure of the daydreaming and imaginal processes. Fairly extensive normative data are available for the scale, which is now widely used. The subject had an "absorption in daydreaming" score of 73, relatively low compared with the college population (M=95, S.D. 18.8) and a positive reaction to daydreaming score of 45, within the normal range (M=39, S.D.=7.3). This finding correlates with some of her verbalizations that she is able to deal with her marital problems through escape into her daydreams.

She scores 37 (in the high normal range) on "Frightened reactions to daydreams" (M=29, S.D.=7.3), indicating that she is very likely to act on her imagination and considers the content of her mental life to be very real. This observation is further supported by the problem solving and daydream score of 44 (M=34, S.D.=7.6), placing her in the high normal range for seeing daydreams as useful to solve problems. Ms. Y. is in the high range of normal on "Bizarre-improbable content" of her daydreams with a score of 36 (M=31, S.D.=8.3). This scale correlates fairly well with obsessional/neurotic trends in daydreaming. The subject is in the upper limits of normal in daydreaming frequency with a score of 43 (M=37, S.D.=8.5). She is relatively low in the fear of failure daydream content at 17 (M=23, S.D.=8.4), and is low normal in hostile daydream content at 24 (M=28, S.D.=9.2). She has an average number of sexual daydreams, scoring a 37, (M=35, S.D.=9.6), and was very low on heroic daydreams (that is, the Walter Mitty variety), with a score of 16 (M=29, S.D.=10.8), reflecting her depression. The most extreme score was that on the self-report tendency item, where she scored 36 (M=4, S.D.=9.6). This scale is specifically designed to tap the degree to which talking about daydreaming is viewed by the respondent as either negative or positive. It is correlated largely with health factors and not with neuroticism or with obsessive-emotional daydream scales. Her high score probably indicates that Ms. Y. counterphobically tends to talk about her inner life in an attempt to deal with some of the anxieties stimulated by her daydreams. Overall, she is not particularly anxious, and is quite accepting of her extremely rich fantasy life and of her tendency to become absorbed in the imagining process.

The Out-of-Body Experience

During a "sound-off" time period, Ms. Y. reported that she was, "calm, just kind of thinking about thoughtful kinds of things, thinking about laughter and life and kind of jumping all around." Then she said, "the noise came on and at first really shocked me, sounded really loud, then I thought the deep noise was like I was in an airplane, and I really got off on this trip, like I was being an airplane and able to fly, and the sound was really relaxing and I just kind of took off." She went on to say "it felt like I was weightless, going through the air, a great feeling, and everything seemed to be going pretty fast." Then, "My mind just took off, I felt comfortable with the sounds." There was a period of fear. She said, "Suddenly I began to wonder what it must have felt like for a guy sitting blindfolded, maybe with sodium pentothal going through him, and really weird things, like death sort of things. Then I thought I'd get off on something else so I had some sexual fantasies going through my head for a while. I couldn't stay on anything very long for a period, and then there were extremely realistic kinds of things, not like fantasies. Then I began to be afraid of where my fantasy was going to take me, and I would try to open my eyes and look around. Although I was calm enough, it seemed like in my mind I was really moving. I felt like I was floating around, just kind of in space, and then at times I felt like I was on some kind of a trip or something." In response to some questioning she then indicated that "my body shook when I was coming out of the tape, like I was cold. It shook like quick jerks."

Although the subject indicated that she had never had out-of-body experiences in the past, two or three days after the session, during an intense daydream, she recalled that as a child, she had suffered sexual and physical abuse from an alcoholic father over a period of years, a fact she had forgotten and about which she felt a great deal of guilt. She said that the sensation she had on the tape, the spinning, the jerking feeling, along with the roaring sound, was very similar to what she felt at the time of that abuse. In fact she used this distancing technique to deal with the strong emotional reactions engendered by the physical and sexual abuse. Her initial reaction to the out-of-body experience was highly positive, which correlates with the fact that she places great emphasis on the positive aspects of daydreaming and fantasy. At some point during the OBE, a variety of frightening fantasy elements intruded into the "reality" of the experience, which she was then able to repress, even within the out-of-body

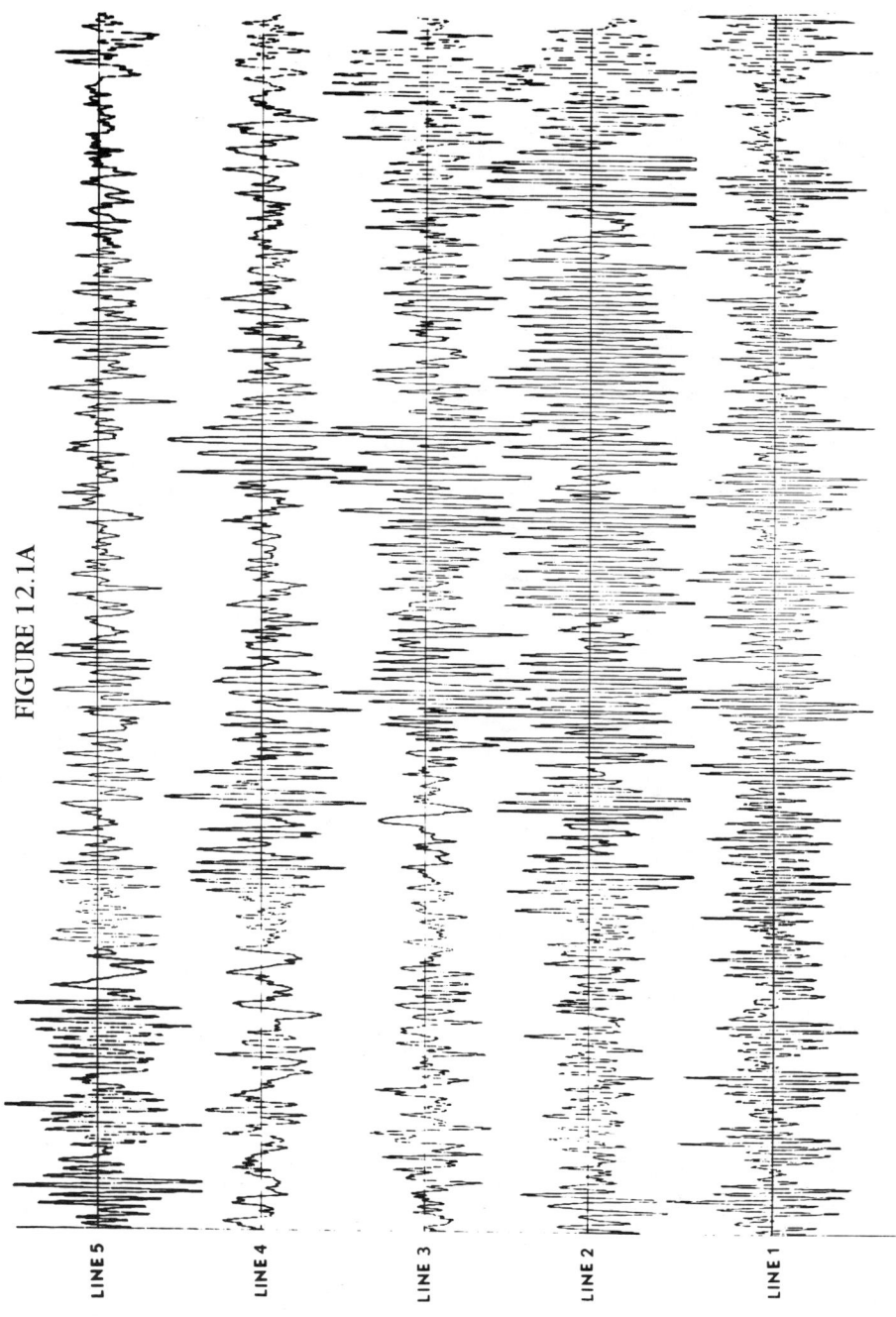

FIGURE 12.1A

FIGURE 12.1B

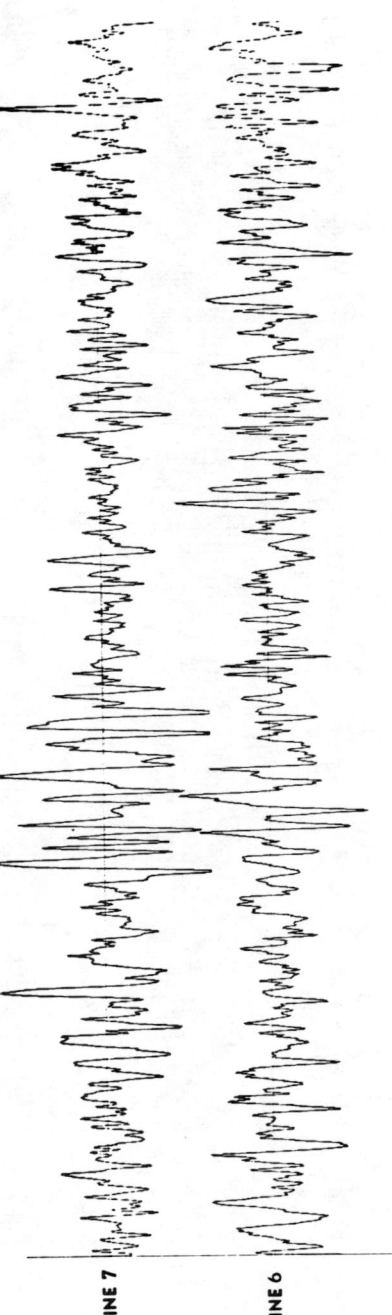

Amplitude vs. Time EEG data. Close to the typical raw clinical EEG. Each line represents 15 seconds of data. The first line is "tape on" typical EEG, progressing to a transition phase in lines 2, 3, 4, and 5, and to Stage 4 sleep in lines 6 and 7. Lines 2, 3, and 4 represent a quasi-Stage 3 sleep variant, the *OBE transition zone.*

FIGURE 12.2A

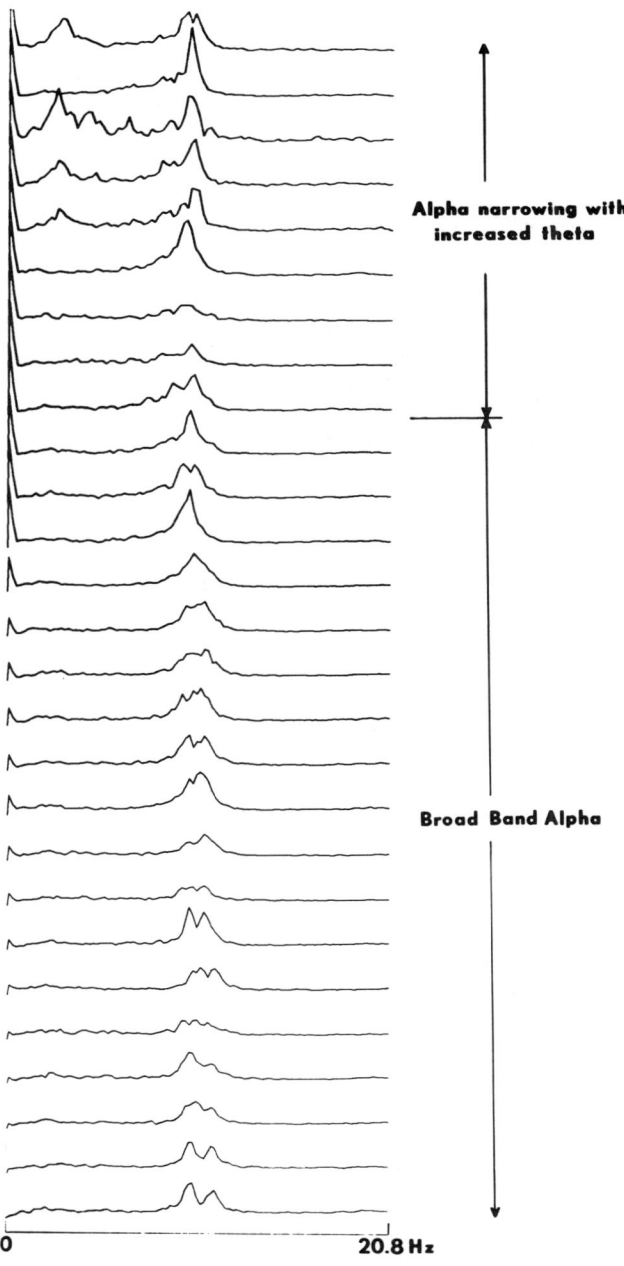

FIGURE 12.2B

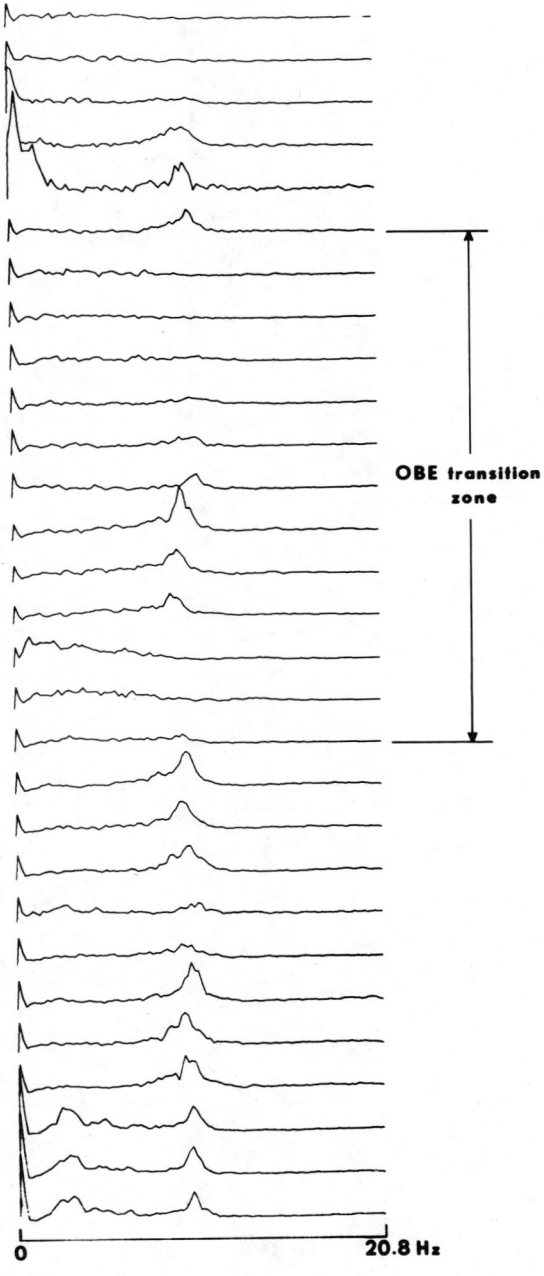

FIGURE 12.2C

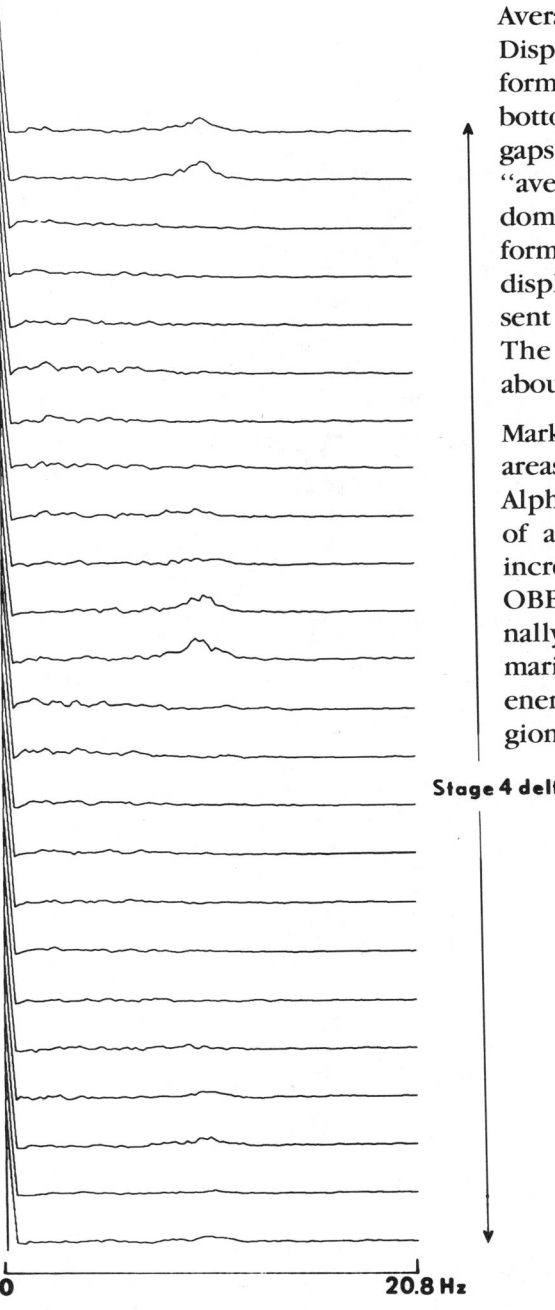

Averages of the Power Spectral Display in simplified graphic form. Time is evolving from bottom to top. Due to time gaps in the recorded data these "averages" in the frequency domain do not represent a uniform number of samples per display line, nor do they represent a uniform time evolution. The averages are usually of about 14 spectra per line.

Marked on these displays are areas representing Broad Band Alpha, a progressive narrowing of alpha frequency band, an increased theta amplitude, the OBE transition zone, and finally, Stage 4 sleep, with primarily delta frequencies and energy concentrated in this region.

FIGURE 12.3

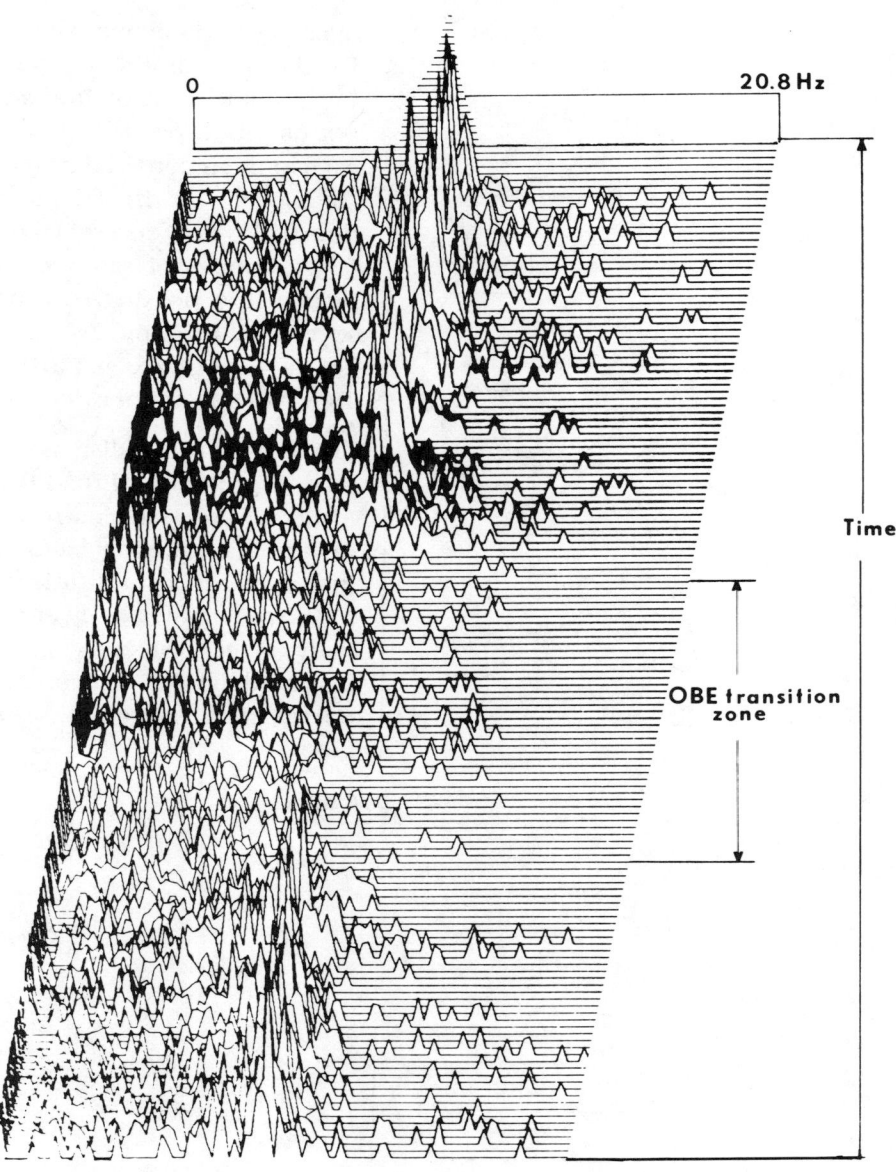

Another Power Spectral Display of the OBE transition zone in a three-dimensional form. The even spread of energy across theta and delta bands with virtually no alpha and no peaks is clearly seen here.

state. It was not until after the tape that the true nature of the disturbing affect was uncovered by a secondarily recalled memory.

Electroencephalographic Findings

One can note in the electroencephalographic chronology shown in Figures 12.1 through Figures 12.3 the following sequence: 1) a relaxation effect as indicated by broad frequency band alpha waves with much reduced beta; 2) a narrowing of the alpha frequency band; 3) an increased theta amplitude; 4) the "OBE wave shape," which has virtually no alpha, but is spread across the theta and delta frequencies, a pattern phenomenologically similar to Stage 3 sleep; and 5) delta (Stage 4) sleep. The tables represent findings in one occipital lead only. The other lead had remarkably similar results; with changes occurring in phase between hemispheres.

It is possible, then, that one difference between those who report out-of-body experiences and those who do not is a conscious awareness of the transition. Thus, the induced out-of-body experience appears to occur in a transitional theta-delta band in the case of Ms. Y., where she retains a greater degree of conscious awareness than is usual for this Stage 3 sleep state. Metaphorically, this represents a possible "window" in consciousness, as though the mind is no longer constrained by the physical location of brain in the cranium since the brain is neither in one state nor in the other.

What, then, are we to make of these findings? Although there is no accurate way of pinpointing exactly when the out-of-body experience occurred, it appears to be clearly related to a final brief sampling interval, and occurred at the end of a "tape on" phase of a session and was accompanied by some rather dramatic, and obvious to the naked eye, changes in the electroencephalographic pattern, as compared with the many previous non-OBE periods over several sessions. The early history of depersonalization episodes in response to abuse by her father is also intriguing. It may well be that such defensive operations employed in the face of extreme trauma may pave the way for subsequent OBEs in adult life since decathexis of the body boundaries had become a familiar and customary means of coping. In Chapter Ten we noted that a whole variety of changes in cathexis of the bodily and mental ego allow one to differentiate a continuum of states from out-of-body experiences on the normal end of the spectrum, to the schizophrenic disintegration and psychedelic drug experiences, on the other end of the spectrum. Thus, it would be reasonable to speculate that the same underlying mechanism that produced Ms. Y.'s unpleasant depersonalization as a child was later transformed to effect this subsequent decathexis of body boundaries, producing the pleasant experience in the laboratory as an adult, which helped her avoid the horrible memory.

The electroencephalographic results are even more interesting. A key to understanding this phenomenon seems to be the notion of a transitional state, or "window," when out-of-body experiences and possibly other unusual states of consciousness might occur. Wilber (1980) describes the phenomenon of bardo, which means gap, transition state, or "in between." Tibetan Monks utilized this concept in an elaborate ritual surrounding death. Using a Buddhist framework, Wilber extends the concept of bardo to describe the gap in between "this moment and the next," (p. 163), as well as between death and rebirth within the Buddhist cultural frame. He states that "what happens at the time of death and birth is what happens between each moment that passes" (p. 163). Thus, the concept of transitional state is pervasive in Buddhist psychology. It has also been postulated to be the origin of various parapsychological phenomena, according to researchers in Soviet Block countries (*Brain/Mind Bulletin*, 1983). They report that "psychic phenomena may occur at the meeting of two states, stress and bodily relaxation" (p. 1). A French researcher, George Clauzure, says that psi functioning takes place in brief dynamic intervals. The two states, he says, each "may contain a window with psi occurring only when the two windows are opposite each other" (p. 1).

These oversimplified metaphors certainly present difficulties in describing these states. Associated metaphors from theoretical physics are only slightly less obscure. A variety of other states similar to out-of-body experience result from the effects of neuroleptic tranquilizers such as haloperidol or chlorpromazine, which can produce alphoid EEG states. Deep coma will also produce high voltage slow waves (Silverman 1963) similar to those seen in this study. A clinical electroencephalographer who saw Ms. Y's EEG said it was similar to an occipital slow wave of sleep variant seen in children, although our subject was not asleep. The occult literature (Fox 1962) describes cataleptic states similar to coma, but none of the literature indicates that such states are absolutely necessary for the out-of-body state. Very deep hypnosis, as reported by Sherman (1972), shows EEG findings similar to those we found with Monroe. Marked amplitude, rather than frequency diminution, was distinguishable by Sherman in the state of very deep hypnosis. This finding could be due to the difficulty in discerning sporadic frequency content when analyzing complex amplitude-time domain data, that is, the wave form appears to change amplitude in groups, which may, in fact, also have frequency shifts.

A variety of psychological states may be related to these transitional phenomena. This concept may be applicable not only to parapsychological experiences, but to a variety of other less unusual altered states of consciousness as well. The notion of transitional state obviates the need to define an absolute and stable neurophysiological state that is specific for the OBE. This point of view is much more in keeping with modern dynamic views both of the mind and of neurophysiology.

Thirteen — THE MIND/BODY TRAP

Up to this point, we have presented varied perspectives on the phenomena of altered mind/body perception. However, we have purposely avoided a detailed consideration of one of the major and most controversial issues in the field. We are, of course, referring to the question—does mind "really" separate from body? Although our focus throughout the book has been psychological, rather than parapsychological, no thoroughgoing discussion of altered mind/body perception would be complete without an examination of this question. Therefore, we will devote our final chapter to this provocative question, although we advise the reader to keep in mind throughout this discourse the caveat suggested many years ago by Emmanuel Kant in *Critique of Pure Reason* (Smith translation):

> To know what question may reasonably be asked is already a great and necessary proof of sagacity and insight. For if the question is absurd in itself and calls for an answer when none is required, it not only brings shame on the preponderer of the question but may betray an incautious listener into absurd answers, thus presenting, as the ancients said, the ludicrous spectacle of one man milking a he-goat and the other holding a sieve underneath (p. 97).

THE SEARCH FOR PROOF

We begin by studying how others have sought to answer this question. The approaches of other investigators to "prove" that mind separates from body can be subdivided into two general categories: 1) laboratory experiments with gifted subjects, and 2) retrospective verifications of out-of-body percepts. Reports from this first category of laboratory investigations have been succinctly summarized by Rogo (1984). These efforts usually involve an experienced out-of-body subject, who is willing to induce an OBE in a laboratory setting and attempt to "travel" into another room or a distant locale, where he or she attempts to affect a detector, which would verify his or her presence. These detectors have varied from instruments to humans and animals. Reports include those from Osis and McCormick (1980) and Morris et al. (1978). This method of researching the separation hypothesis, the favorite of the parapsychologist, has produced mixed results. Instrumental detectors, pet animals of gifted subjects, and human detectors, who are usually psychics, have all been used with some success, responding with various reactions at roughly the same time the gifted subject reports he is in his out-of-body state. The results are neither consistent nor conclusive, however (Blackmore 1984).

The second approach designed to demonstrate that the mind "really" separates from the body often occurs as an afterthought following a spontaneous out-of-body or near-death experience. The effort here is to verify that a perception from the out-of-body state was accurate and could have been perceived in no other manner. This is Sabom's (1982) method in his retrospective reconstructions of NDEs. This approach is also the one favored by theosophists, such as Muldoon and Carrington (1977) and Fox (1962). Monroe (1977) reports an episode in which he pinched an acquaintance of his while he was having an out-of-body experience and subsequently verified the pinch by observing a bruise on the skin of the person he had pinched. From the hundreds of OBE reports we have examined, it is obvious that this method is one that is commonly applied by the naive subject, who wishes to determine after his OBE if he was "really out."

These approaches to the question have failed to prove conclusively that mind separates from body. The investigators themselves, in most cases, will be the first ones to acknowledge the inconclusiveness of the results. The two methods are thought to be inadequate for a variety of reasons. We will briefly classify and review four criticisms.

1. *Alternative paranormal explanations*. This problem with efforts to prove separation is frequently pointed out by the parapsy-

chologists themselves. If a gifted subject influences an instrument detector in a different room, this finding does not require actual separation of mind from body to explain it. The subject may simply have influenced the detector through psychokinesis. Similarly, if a perception of a distant event occurs during an out-of-body experience and that event is subsequently verified to have occurred at the time of the OBE, the knowledge of the event can be explained on the basis of telepathy or clairvoyance. The postulation of a perceiving mind floating in a physical location separate from the body is again not a necessary assumption to make sense out of the findings.

2. *Alternative natural explanations.* Singer (1981) points out that our everyday intuitions are notoriously unreliable. We are poor observers and catalogers of our natural environment. We seriously underestimate the probability of rare events or "coincidences." In fact the mathematical probabilities of rare events often run counter to intuition. If someone is asked, for example, about the probability of at least two people in a class of 30 students having the same birthday, most people will estimate the odds to be approximately one in a thousand. We are shocked to hear that the chances are seven out of ten. Singer notes that we are apt to conclude, uncritically and immediately, that a mysterious event reflects a mysterious cause and to overlook ordinary causes simply because the event is not generally associated with ordinary causes. Whether or not clairvoyant dreams occur, for instance, one can nevertheless expect a dramatic correspondence of a dream with a real life event several times during one's lifetime based on chance alone.

From the perspective of Singer, Sabom's (1982) data on the "extrabodily" perceptions of NDE subjects are highly suspect. He would point out that only 32 of Sabom's 116 subjects reported that they could observe events during their own resuscitations. Of these 32, 26 reported general and nonspecific observations, which did not allow for any retrospective verification. Only six of the 32 reported observations in sufficient detail to permit some subsequent validation. The probabilities involved in such reports are difficult to figure, but Singer might very well propose that chance alone could explain these findings.

3. *Methodological and design errors.* The foregoing discussion of Sabom's work leads us directly into this third area of criticism about such approaches. Even though a control group of cardiac patients who had not had NDEs were found by Sabom to be unable to imagine resuscitation procedures with comparable accuracy, the

control subjects did not have the same sensory (mainly auditory) information available as compared to subjects who were truly resuscitated (Blackmore 1984). In the laboratory investigations a recurrent methodological problem is knowing with certainty that the detector is reacting at the same moment in which the subject is "out of body." The researcher must be content that the two events occur roughly at the same time. One could go on at some length cataloging the methodological and design problems with the experimental investigations reported.

4. *Discrediting the researcher.* This method of debunking the reports emanating from the two preceding appoaches ordinarily takes two forms: the investigator is naive, gullible, and highly biased, or the researcher is fraudulent. An example of the former is Gardner's (1981) commentary on Professor John G. Taylor's work on metal bending. Taylor, a brilliant mathematician, was enthralled with the psychic Uri Geller and uncritically accepted all his claims. An example of the latter is reported by Rogo (1978) in a book on out-of-body experience. He reports that David Black tried to pin down Robert Monroe on some of the details of his out-of-body travels, only to find Monroe lacking in recall. Black hinted that Monroe may have invented some of his OBE accounts.

After this concise cataloging of commonly leveled criticisms, we will discuss at length two more fundamental and interrelated problems with these efforts to prove separation of mind from body: 1) the assumption of an "objective" reality superior to "subjective" reality that can be experimentally verified; and 2) the philosophical assumptions inherent in the search for mind within the body, or, as philosophers often put it, the "ghost in the machine."

REALITY AS PARTICIPATORY

We begin our discussion of the first problem by looking at the nature of reality in the out-of-body experience. A cursory reading of OBE reports in the literature will leave the reader with the distinct impression that reality in the OBE is represented on a continuum from totally unlike the physical environment to more or less identical with it. On the former end of the continuum are subjects such as Fox (1962), who reports encounters with entities and locales that are completely unlike the environment in which the physical body remains. At the other end of the continuum, we have the reports of mundane OBEs, such as Mr. A. in Chapter One, who seemingly perceived the environment of his bedroom as he perceived it during ordinary waking consciousness. At a middle point in the continuum, we have researchers such as Blackmore (1984), who asserts that the reality perceived during an OBE is an imaginary one based on a "cognitive map" of what the surrounding environment looks like. She describes OBE perception as an approximation of the physical environment. This view is similar to ours and to that of Professor Arthur Ellison (1979), who describes his own OBE perceptions as corresponding closely to the environment of his physical body, but differing slightly in some minor points. For example he reported an OBE to us that was characterized by an accurate visualization of his bedroom except for the presence of a laundry basket on the floor. After his out-of-body experience, he noted that there was, in fact, no laundry basket in his room. As Blackmore (1984) points out, one of the few things we know for sure about OBE percepts is that they are often erroneous. Whether they are accurate is much more controversial.

Clearly, different OBE subjects perceive different versions of reality. How do we account for these discrepancies in reports? The compelling conclusion from these differences is not that there are a number of "objective" realities, but that the subjective participation of the OBE subject in the creation of his or her own percept is the primary determinant of the nature of reality in the out-of-body experience. This conclusion leads us to a discussion focused on the nature of reality in general.

With the discoveries of quantum physics, the notion of an "objective" reality "out there," independent of the observer's input, is increasingly untenable. The universe we find depends on the questions we ask of it. Reality is a participatory experience in which the perceiver determines to a large extent the nature of his or her own perceptions. This point of view is strongly supported by Polanyi (1965) and is also compatible with the psychoanalytic perspective. In the analytic situation the perception of the analyst is colored by the analysand's wishes, fears, preexisting beliefs, attitudes, prejudices, fantasies, and past experiences with similar figures. The concept of transference in psychoanalysis is based on the premise that one's experience of the analyst is based on one's subjective experiences of similar figures in the past. We attribute to him or her qualities of these figures that come from our own unconscious, and the assumptions we form about the analyst cause us to scotomize certain sensory data about him or her and overvalue other data.

Transference is a pervasive phenomenon that extends beyond the analytic situation to relationships in general. Every perception of another person in a relationship is a mixture of "real" observations and transference. Similarly, what we perceive as reality is essentially a transference reality, a personal construct, based on a combination of subjective factors and objective sensory data. This participatory reality is determined principally by four interrelated elements: 1) the observer's belief system, 2) the observer's state of consciousness, 3) the explanatory usefulness of the percept, and 4) the observer's narcissistic investment in a particular paradigm. Let us briefly examine these four determinants.

1. *Belief system.* We are not likely to see that in which we do not believe. In psychoanalysis that which is repressed, and therefore unconscious, is not part of one's personal reality. In fact certain unacceptable wishes and feelings are repressed for the very purpose of making them nonexistent, that is, not real, as far as the individual involved in the act of repression is concerned. This process goes on at an unconscious level as a kind of automatic censor. We know, however, that the repressed material can be brought into consciousness through the process of free association, dream analysis, and interpretation of transference and resistance. As a result of analysis, one can develop an expanded view of his or her own reality. Prior to analysis, if the analysand is told that it is a universal wish to kill off one's father in order to have one's mother to oneself, one may find such a notion preposterous and outrageous. However, following one's own personal analysis, one is likely to accept such an interpretation of reality as quite accurate, since it is now part of one's own personal belief system based on one's own direct experience. The oedipus complex has now been realized, that is, made real, at a personal level so that it has become integrated into one's belief system. Subsequent to analysis, if the analysand attends a production of *Hamlet*, he is likely to see oedipal determinants of Hamlet's dilemma that were not perceived when he saw the play prior to his analysis, since this order of reality was not part of his world view or of his view of himself.

2. *State of consciousness.* Lest we sound as though we are taking an extreme position in asserting that so-called external reality is more or less a construct of the mind, we should clarify that we are

not saying that there are no consensually validated objective aspects of nature. The world of appearances is certainly real. What we are stating is that it is not the only possible or valid reality. It is simply one order of reality among many other possible realities. Moreover, the world of appearances "appears" in a variety of ways depending upon the observer. What we identify as reality tends to be limited by the limitations of our consciousness. Besides the dramatic role that personal belief systems play in defining reality, the state of consciousness of the individual at the time he or she is perceiving is seen by some investigators to be of equal importance. We share the viewpoint of Tart (1972), who proposes the development of what he calls "state specific" sciences. He suggests that different scientific paradigms are needed for the understanding of different phenomena observed during altered states of consciousness, such as hypnosis, meditation, or religious experience. The experience of synesthesia, for example, is for most observers an inference obtained from the reports of other persons, but it is real data of observation only for a person who has experienced it personally from LSD ingestion or similar mind alteration. On a more mundane level, we are all in various arousal levels during the day as influenced by the basic rest and activity cycle, nicotine, caffeine, various over-the-counter remedies, and shifts in attentional focus. These small variations in the state of consciousness affect perception as well. If we apply this point of view to the "reality" of the out-of-body experience, we can postulate that such an experience is only accessible to the subject in a specific altered state of consciousness. More specifically, for disengagement of the mental ego cathexis and the bodily ego cathexis to occur, it is necessary for there to be a preexisting altered state of consciousness characterized by mental calmness, physical relaxation, decreased external sensory input, and diminished internal proprioceptive input.

3. *Explanatory usefulness of the percept.* Another factor that influences the perception of sensory data is its explanatory usefulness. For years scientists have been accused of selecting data, that is, only attending to or reporting that data that can explain the phenomena being studied. Data that confound or complicate the explanation may be unconsciously scotomized. A striking confirmation of this notion comes from Rosenthal (1977), who notes that when an experimenter error occurs, it is almost always in the direction of confirming the experimenter's hypothesis. George Klein (1973) points out that we look for "coherences" in what we perceive to

make the percept understandable. We look for clues, in other words, to explain the "reason" for the event or experience we call reality. As he puts it, "We make an occurrence reasonable by explaining it. In this sense the coherence that we call a 'chair' is actually less real for the microphysicist than is its atomic structure, for 'chair' as an object to sit on has little pertinence to the physicist's domain of variables" (p. 118).

4. *Narcissistic investment in a particular paradigm.* Rothstein (1980) notes that we are all narcissistically invested in a particular paradigm of scientific thought that we embrace as correct and useful. The fervent belief in this paradigm gives us an illusion of having a conceptual framework that will explain all the phenomena that we are likely to encounter in nature. Hence, it assuages our sense of vulnerability and helplessness in the face of a complex universe. Einstein's paradigm has become narcissistically invested by a great many physicists, for example. His theory of relativity provides a coherent understanding of a complex and mysterious external world. Data at odds with the paradigm of Einstein are sometimes not welcomed by the scientific establishment, as demonstrated by the recent newspaper accounts of physicist Henry Hill's attempts to challenge the theory of relativity. Hill was unable to find anyone who would publish his controversial paper and received a "confrontation" by the New York Academy of Sciences. Einstein has become something of a transference figure, resulting in the suspension of rational thinking in some of his adherents, so that all of his discoveries, even highly technical ones, become invested with magic and authority that brook no disagreement.

When the scientist is confronted with new observations or fresh data, he or she will often seize on those aspects that confirm his or her narcissistically invested paradigm and discard or fail to notice those aspects that question the paradigm. Trefil (1983) studied the rejection of scientific claims. He concludes that for claims involving a single statistically insignificant event, scientists tend to reject such claims if alternative explanations exist, even if the probability of these alternative explanations is in the range of 10^{-9} to 10^{-12}. Even if no alternative explanations exist, a claim is often placed in a kind of scientific limbo if it raises serious theoretical inconsistencies. Moreover, a scenario of "statistical fluctuations" is often employed to reject claims originating from statistically insignificant events. Hence, scientists tend to reject claims as anomalous or "noise" when they are incompatible with existing narcissistically invested paradigms.

In the area of OBE research a recent example of this may be found in a report by Salley (1982), which correlates OBE states with REM sleep. Salley argues his case based on one experimental subject and a selective review of the literature. To make his point, he is forced to ignore a number of other contradictory reports in the literature, as though they do not exist.

Having summarized these four determinants of participatory reality, we feel it is appropriate to note the extent to which Western science is preoccupied with ideal states. We are prone to conceptualize perfect states that cannot and do not exist. "Objective" reality may be one such state that is held up by science as an ideal. Erikson (1962) defines reality as a phenomenologically describable world, free from personalized distortion and consensually validated. He contrasts reality with actuality, which he sees as a participatory experience characterized by mutual activation between perceiver and percept. He implies an artificial separation of the percept from the perceiver of it, in his notion of reality, implying that a process akin to phenomenological reduction would bring to light what is "really real," that is, the elements not distorted by personal idiosyncratic projections. It is our view that such a reduced or bracketed reality is not reality at all, but a nonexistent, idealized construct of a particular philosophy of knowledge. Erikson's concept of actuality comes closer to our view of reality, which requires a quasi-empathic step of observer participation in perception.

The efforts of experimental investigators to prove the separation of mind from body are anchored in the assumption that there is an "objective" reality to these experiences, which can be demonstrated and repeated in the laboratory. As we have noted, the results are inconclusive and unconvincing, failing to prove separation even to the parapsychologists, let alone to the skeptical debunkers. Experimental attempts to document paranormal events raise the specter of a powerful and perhaps insurmountable problem in this kind of research. We are referring to the problem of experimenter bias, or the influence of the experimenter on the outcome of his or her experiment. This concept embraces all four of the determinants of reality as we have defined them above.

Rosenthal (1977) has done seminal work in this area. His findings shatter our smugness concerning the purity of the scientific method. He demonstrates that even in the apparently objective context of scientific experimentation, the experimenters' beliefs and expectations concerning the experiment significantly influence the "reality" of the outcome. Twelve experimenters were each given five rats that were to be taught to run a maze with the aid of visual cues. Half of the experimenters were told that the rats had been specially bred for maze brightness while half were told the rats had been bred for maze dullness. Actually, there were no differences between the rats assigned to each of the two groups. At the end of the experiment, the results were clear. The rats that had been run by experimenters expecting brighter behaviors showed significantly superior learning compared to rats run by experimenters expecting dull behavior. If self-fulfilling prophecy and experimenter expectation has such a powerful influence on research with rats, what are the implications for human subjects? In another study by Rosenthal, within each of 18 classrooms an average of 20 percent of the children were reported to classroom teachers as showing unusual potential for intellectual gains. Eight months later these "unusual" children, who had actually been selected at random, showed significantly greater gains in I.Q. than the remaining children in the control group. Clearly, the expectancy of the teachers had powerful effects on the students' performance.

Inglis (1983), an articulate spokesman from the parapsychological perspective, has noted this experimenter effect and cites it as a major determinant of one of the ongoing weaknesses in parapsychological research—the repeatability of experiments. He even suggests that all the efforts of parapsychologists to prove paranormal effects to the greater scientific community may be jeopardized by this factor. He comments on the decline effect, a variation of experimenter bias; and he reports an even more striking example than those of Rosenthal. Professor Neal Miller of the Rockefeller University in New York published groundbreaking work with autonomic nervous system control in rats in 1959. He demonstrated in the laboratory that rats could learn to alter their heartbeats, their blood pressures, their visceral responses, and even the temperature of their ears so that one ear would "blush." As improbable as this early biofeedback work sounds, other researchers obtained the same results using the same technique. Much to Miller's chagrin, he was unable to repeat these experiments four years later, despite the fact that the results had been demonstrated by six different experiments. On examining his series of studies, a picture of progressive decline emerged. Inglis reports a similar problem in the work of Sabin, who following his triumph with the polio vaccine, produced what appeared to be conclusive evidence that herpes virus is a cause of many human cancers. Unfortunately, he had to admit that he was unable to replicate his initial results. This decline effect is also prominent in psychopharmacology research, where new medications may show remarkable results initially, only to lead to disappointment as their use is increased.

Inglis elaborates this problem from the standpoint of unconscious skepticism that may erode the initial enthusiasm for the results. He refers to the Nobel prize winner Charles Richet, who contrasted his initial certainty of and excitement with a parapsychological discovery with the subsequent erosion of his own enthusiasm when he had time to reflect in the privacy of his own mind on the credibility and logic of his results. One begins to question whether such an outcome is real or illusory and whether one has been deceived. This secret skepticism, in Inglis' view, may account for this decline effect. He expands his ideas even further to include a "witness-effect," in which he postulates that certain paranormal effects can be impossible when a skeptical witness is present, and a "location-effect," a label for a well-known phenomenon, that is, the inability of psychics to perform in laboratories or other settings away from home.

This discussion of experimenter influence completes our examination of the first major problem with the efforts to prove separation of mind from body. The "reality" of the out-of-body state is not real in any "objective" sense that will ever likely be demonstrated in a laboratory. It is real to the OBE subject in a powerful and persuasive subjective sense. This fact is most interesting to us and serves to explain partially why we are more interested in the psychology of the phenomena rather than in the objective demonstration of separation of mind from body. We now turn to a consideration of the second major problem with these investigations, which will take us on a brief excursion into philosophy.

THE GHOST IN THE MACHINE

Andre Tardieu once said, "The difficulties lie in our habits of thought rather than in the nature of things." It is just such difficulties that form the basis for the second major problem with investigations designed to prove that mind separates from body. We view the concept of mind as a habit of thought, a construct of language that reassures us that we are more than our brains, more than our physical bodies. The central philosophical problem in asking whether mind "really" separates from body is the assumption that mind is a measurable substance different from brain, rather than a figure of speech or a creation borne of man's ability to reflect on himself. This mind/body dichotomy is a conceptual trap, which has a long history in philosophy. This philosophical search for the "ghost in the machine" is often referred to as the dualistic viewpoint, and it postulates that there are two principles: matter and spirit. Thinking in dualistic terms is a fundamentally human phenomenon. A moment's reflection produces numerous examples of this habit of thought: right and left hemisphere, yin and yang, animus and anima, love and hate, good and bad, positive and negative charges of electricity, and so forth.

It was not until René Descartes (1596-1650) that dualism received its formal elaboration in modern philosophical terms. His famous "cogito ergo sum" (I think, therefore I am) implies that personal consciousness is the only sure knowledge that an individual has. Consciousness itself is identified with spirit, which was to him a substance as real and concrete as a substance he called body or matter. In Cartesian terms body was defined as extended, space-filling physical material and mind as "thinking thing" (res cogitans), which was unextended, that is, not space-filling and purely spiritual. Moreover, Descartes postulated that these two principles mutually influence each other, resulting in the position known as interactionism. Subsequent to Descartes' contributions, Leibnitz (1646-1716) suggested another dualistic theory, which he termed parallelism. In Leibnitz' conceptualization, mind and body are perfectly correlated but do not interact with one another or influence one another in any way. Sulloway (1980) and Edelheit (1976) have suggested that this psychophysical parallelism, in nonmetaphysical form, served as an important basis for the evolution of Freudian psychoanalytic thinking.

The most extreme and most contemporary example of psychophysical parallelism is in the extraordinary partnership of the neurophysiologist Eccles and the philosopher Popper (1977), who not only assert that mind is separate from body, but even claim to have identified the location of mind in a layer of neocortex! In an address to the American Parapsychological Association (1977), Eccles referred to his position as, "a stronger dualism than before because we insist in the first place that the mind is over and above the brain and that all our ideas are in the mind before they are in the brain; they only come into the brain when we make them into language and thoughts and intentions" (pp. 261-62). This extreme position, largely unsupported, provides a deceptively simple solution to the out-of-body problem. The mind simply lies on top of matter and hence can be separated from it!

The dualistic viewpoint holds enormous appeal because of the implication that a soul, immortal and indestructible, lies within the physical body and is released at the moment of death. The *Oxford Dictionary of English Etymology* (1966) indicates that soul, psyche, and mind have identical etymological origins. There is little doubt that the out-of-body experience has attracted the interest of reputable scientific investigators as well as the general public, not simply because of some fascination with altered states of consciousness, but because of the possibility that the OBE represents a living model of what may well happen after the physical body dies. The search for the "ghost in the machine"—whether it be in the OBE laboratory experiment, in the philosopher's treatise, or in the front pew of the corner church—is related to the pervasive human wish to survive death. Becker (1973) notes that the terror of death is the fundamental anxiety of humans. The central existential problem of humankind is to come to terms with this terror. Hence, immortality ideologies and myths of heroic transcendence are fundamental to all civilizations.

Becker poignantly describes the existential paradox of the human condition: "He (man) is out of nature and hopelessly in it; he is dual, up in the stars and yet housed in a heart-pumping, breath-gasping body that once belonged to fish and still carries the gill marks to prove it...he has an awareness of his own splendid uniqueness in that he sticks out of nature with a towering majesty, and yet he goes back into the ground a few feet in order blindly and dumbly to rot and disappear forever. It is a terrifying dilemma to be in and to have to live with" (p. 26). The dualistic perspective is appealing because it serves as a partial antidote to the sobering possibility that humans are simply way stations on the inexorable Darwinian path of evolution. Unfortunately, at this way station the species has developed sufficiently to possess a conscious awareness of its own death and decay. Humans have emerged from the instinctual, nonreflective lower animals but have been given consciousness of their own uniqueness and their own individuality. The existential terror in acknowledging the benign indifference of the universe is simply too dreadful to face. Humans need illusion. They need to deny their essential "creatureliness." No matter how illogical and no matter how impossible and unprovable, humans need to believe in the mind/body trap.

A PHILOSOPHICAL PERSPECTIVE ON THE OBE

If, as we have suggested, the dualistic perspective is problematic in understanding the out-of-body experience, are there other philosophical points of view which may be useful? Descriptions of OBEs raise three primary issues: 1) the spatial perspective is altered so that the individual experiences himself or herself as outside his normal perceived location in the body, 2) the OBE subject feels a sense that he or she is a complete person in all aspects in this new location, and 3) the experience is life-changing, highly positive, and integrating. Few philosophers have addressed these issues. Grosso (1976) proposes that we have developed an erroneous mode of thinking about consciousness. He says it is misleading to think that consciousness in some sense is located in the body and somehow manages to get out of the body under conditions of OBE or NDE. He suggests that it may be "more in accord with the truth to think of the body as located in the field of consiousness" (p. 180). He refers to this metaphoric position as hypophenomenalism.

The philosophical perspective, which, in our opinion, has more heuristic value as a model for understanding the out-of-body experience is one that is identified with monism, the complementary trend within philosophy to dualistic thinking. Whereas dualism asserts that there are two principles, monism rests on the assumption of one basic principle. This principle may be spirit, in keeping with Buddhist doctrine, or it may be viewed as matter, a form of nonmetaphysical monism consistent with the thinking of Feigl's (1975) identity thesis. Influenced by Feigl, Globus (1973a, 1973b, 1980) has developed a theory of structural identity that is useful for our purposes. He argues in favor of a monistic ontology whose fundamental elements are neither mental nor physical, but simply structural. This common structure varies with the position of the observer, so that Globus views the concepts of mental and physical as related to different ways of knowing the common structure depending on one's perspective. A scientific observer may maintain a subject-object distinction, while a meditator, on the other hand, dissolves that distinction, along with the observing part of himself or herself that serves the function of self-awareness. Hence, the nature of knowledge, in his or her view, varies as a function of our manner of acquaintance with it. This notion is similar to our concept of participatory reality advanced earlier in this chapter.

The classical identity thesis, in its simplist form, states that consciousness is identical with neural events. Identity theory, then, can account for the private "subjective" events as opposed to the public "objective" events of consciousness quite easily. In our view the fundamental distinction is between the actual representation of events as thoughts with concrete content and the nonspecific systems that are concerned with levels of awareness, that is, the context within which thinking occurs. To use the ground-figure analogy, this nonrepresentational context is essentially the ground while the representational thought content is the figure. The neural context is not the result of external input but is simply intrinsic neural events (neurochemical, neurophysiological, and neuroanatomical elements) acted upon by representational events, that is, thought content. To summarize, representational events are identical with the content of conscious thoughts, whereas nonrepresentational events are identical with the neuronal substrate, which is the consciousness of the thought. Altered states of consciousness, then, are clearly examples of alterations in the nonrepresentational neural context rather than in the thought itself, although this context has a potentially important impact on the private and public components of thought. This distinction helps to explain Tart's (1972) state specific theory of scientific knowledge. Colors look different when one is on LSD largely because the neural context is altered, not because of any alteration in the mental content itself, thus providing a different substrate in which the perception takes place.

Applying these ideas to the specific altered state of consciousness known as the out-of-body experience requires us to pinpoint more precisely the nature of the "phenomenal I," that is, the experience of oneself. This "I" is the observer of thought content and is therefore nonrepresentational. As this "I," this experience of oneself, is context rather than content, nonrepresentational rather than representational, it is not delimited, as thought content is. In other words it is boundariless from a spatial perspective. While one maintains mental self-representations that are delimited, the observer of these mental representations is not. This experiencer or observer that we call "I" is, of course, composed of brain elements. We conceptualize the OBE within this model as an attentional shift from the thought content to the nonrepresentational "I," or, in other words, from the thought to the thinker. If the neural context within the out-of-body state continues to be nonrepresentational, the OBE may be experienced as no more than a disembodied point of consciousness, as was the case in 24 percent of our subjects. However, as is more commonly the case, the nonrepresentational state provides a striking paradigm clash, resulting in the restitutive elaboration of the body scheme fully cathected with bodily ego cathexis.

This shift in attention from thought content to thinker is also a primary characteristic of the mental posture associated with both the concentrative and the mindfulness meditative traditions (Maliszewski et al. 1981; Brown 1977). Twenty-seven percent of our OBE sample were meditating just prior to their OBEs. Moreover, out-of-body experiences are commonly reported in the early stages of meditation. In most descriptions of meditation, the effects of the process are described in glowing terms not dissimilar to those applied to out-of-body experiences, which seem to involve similar attentional alterations. Hence, one could speculate that the remarkable integrating effect often reported in connection with out-of-body experiences is very likely a result of this particular attentional shift and is therefore not necessarily unique to the OBE. A testable hypothesis for future research would be that such mystical-integrative experiences result primarily from such a change in attention.

The emotional reaction is a matter of psychology rather than philosophy. However, it should be noted that there is a fundamental similarity, affectively and phenomenologically, between the experience of one's self as a point of consciousness, that is, the nonrepresentational "I" described by many of our OBE subjects, and the experience of unifying and limitless pure consciousness supposedly associated with popular meditative strategies such as Transcendental Meditation. This "nonattachment" to thought content is seen in virtually all meditative traditions as a primary cognitive mechanism for successful meditation, although why the shift should produce such a startling response is not at all clear, suggesting the need for further research efforts.

At this point in our discussion of the question—does mind "really" separate from the body—it occurs to us that there are three possibilities: 1) there is an answer, but scientists are unable to find the answer; 2) the question is meaningless and therefore should be discarded; or 3) the question is unanswerable when phrased in dualistic terminology, but could be answered, theoretically, if properly rephrased and approached in more acceptable conceptual terms.

We favor the second possibility, that is, that the question is inherently absurd. Our study of this problem leads us to conclude that we have happened upon a Kantian question in which we have one man milking a he-goat and the other holding a sieve underneath.

CONCLUSION

Having examined the separation question, it may be useful to summarize our understanding of the out-of-body experience. Our model, which may be called the ego uncoupling model, assumes that an altered state of consciousness unlike the usual alert, waking, rational, problem-solving state, is a necessary context for these experiences to occur. In this altered state, in which there is mental calmness and physical relaxation, sensory input from external sources and the proprioceptive input from internal sources diminish in importance and receive less attention cathexis. The out-of-body experience begins when the cathexis is withdrawn from the bodily ego and a dissociation, or uncoupling, between the bodily ego and the mental ego occurs. When the subject has a sensation that his or her mind is disconnected from his or her body, there is a perceptual restitutive effect to try to make internal sense out of what is going on. The body scheme is reinvested with cathexis so that the subject feels whole, and internal images of what would ordinarily be seen if one were looking from the vantage point of being "outside the body" are evoked. These internal images, which are approximations of the actual environment, are viewed as real. Horowitz (1983) notes that undercontrol of the usual sensory and perceptual processes, which is characteristic of this form of altered state of consciousness, results in the unplanned emergence of images. This spontaneous and unexpected appearance of these images contributes to a sense of their estrangement from thoughtlike domains of meaning and gives them a quasi-perceptual quality. These internal images reign supreme as a result of the relatively quiescent external sensory input during the experience. What is most adaptive under the circumstances may be to disregard established conventions of the nature of reality and accept fabrications as if they were real in the service of making internal sense of an unusual experience and in keeping with the need to believe in a dualistic framework.

The altered state of consciousness in which the uncoupling of the bodily ego and the mental ego takes place seems to be correlated with electroencephalographic findings that suggest a transitional neurophysiological state between stable electroencephalographic patterns. Whether the neurophysiological changes precede and contribute to the causation of the OBE or simply follow and result from the OBE is not clear. What is clear is that the uncoupling of the bodily ego and the mental ego is the final common pathway of many different causative factors. Given the appropriate context of the altered state of consciousness described previously, any number of stimuli may work alone or in concert to produce the uncoupling. These stimuli include a variety of unconscious psychological issues that may come together in an overdetermined fashion to produce a separation experience with multilayered meanings. The physiological factor of decreased proprioceptive signals may in and of itself be sufficient to cause the uncoupling. Cardiac arrest may produce another physiological stimulus for the dissociation of bodily ego and mental ego. We are aware of one case in which a young man's temporal lobe seizures were heralded by an aura involving an out-of-body experience, indicating that neurophysiological changes in the cortex can in some instances produce the same effect. Migraine auras may produce similar results. Finally, drugs such as hallucinogens, alpha-methyldopa, and haloperidol (Lukianowicz 1967) also have been reported to precipitate the uncoupling characteristic of OBE, apparently on a biochemical basis.

This ego-uncoupling model is an integrative one that acknowledges the complexity of the phenomenon and allows for multifaceted contributions to the final common pathway. It also attempts to put to rest the assumption of mind as a substance or thing that can be disconnected from brain yet maintain highly complex perceptual and cognitive functions. However, it is also a model that eschews the notion that the OBE is an hallucination of a diseased mind. The evidence simply does not support that conclusion. As Stevenson (1983) points out, many persons who are not mentally ill have unshared sensory experiences. Unlike hallucinations, the spontaneous OBE is an isolated event that is not related to any illness or known disturbance and not associated with generalized loss of contact with one's surroundings. Stevenson cautions us that the lumping together of all unshared sensory experiences as pathological hallucinations may actually prevent people from reporting or even experiencing phenomena such as the OBE. It is incumbent upon us as psychiatrists to be open to the full range and breadth of human experience in such a way that we differentiate disintegrating and pathological experiences from integrating and creative ones. With its power to judge and label human experience, psychiatry has historically found itself in the midst of a dialectical struggle between being a repressive force that limits and perpetuates culture and a creative force that expands it.

We have now examined the OBE from the standpoint of metapsychology, from the psychoanalytic vantage point of determinants and meanings, from the neurophysiological point of view, and from a philosophical perspective. Despite this attempt at a comprehensive analysis, we are left with the distinct feeling that much is unsettled and perhaps more questions have been raised than answers provided. Given the current state of scholarship in this area, all explanations must be partial and incomplete to some extent. We leave the reader with some reflections of Allen Wheelis (1980):

> Consciousness is a flame, bright, waivering, hot; is fragile, can be snuffed out. As flame is tied to candle so consciousness is tied to body; no more can consciousness survive the body's death than flame the candle's being used up. The question is: Must the 'I' be lodged in that individual flame or may it escape to find a home in illumination at large? Must all value lie in the transient flame which, as it well knows, is for the most part miserable and petty? Cannot the flame love illumination more than it loves itself? Can one identify the 'I' with life beyond the self? (pp. 176-77)

BIBLIOGRAPHY

CHAPTER ONE

Blackmore, S.J. 1984. "A Postal Survey of OBE's and Other Experiences." *Journal of the Society for Psychical Research* 52(796):225–44.
———. 1982. "Have You Ever Had an OBE?: The Wording of the Question." *Journal of the Society for Psychical Research* 51(791):292–302.
———. 1978. "Parapsychology and Out-of-the-Body Experiences." *Perspectives in Parapsychology I*. London: Transpersonal Books/Society for Psychical Research, pp. 5–33.
Broad, C.D. 1966. *Lectures on Psychical Research*. London: Routledge and Kegan, Paul: The Humanities Press.
Crookall, R. 1965. *Intimations of Immortality*. London: James Clarke and Co. Ltd.
———. 1960. *The Study and Practice of Astral Projection*. New Hyde Park, NY: University Books, Inc.
Eastman, M. 1962. "Out-of-the-Body Experiences." *Proceedings of the American Society for Psychical Research* 53(193):287–309.
Ehrenwald, J. 1974. "Out-of-the-Body Experiences and the Denial of Death." *Journal of Nervous and Mental Disease* 159(4):227–33.
Fox, O. (pseudonym). 1962. *Astral Projection: A Record of Out-of-the-Body Experiences*. Secaucus, NJ: University Books (originally published in 1939).
Green, C.E. 1968. *Out-of-the-Body Experiences*. London: Hamish Hamilton.
———. 1967. "Ecsomatic Experiences and Related Phenomena." *Journal of the Society for Psychical Research* 44(733):111–30.
Haraldsson, E., A. Gudmundsdottir, J.L. Ragnarsson, and S. Jonsson. 1977. "National Survey of Psychical Experiences and Attitudes Towards the Paranormal in Iceland." *Research in Parapsychology—1976*. Metuchen, NJ: Scarecrow Press, pp. 182–86.
Hart, H. 1954. "ESP Projection: Spontaneous Cases and the Experimental Method." *The Journal of the American Society for Psychical Research* XLVIII (4):121–46.
Hill, J.A. 1918. *Man Is a Spirit*. New York: Doran.
Irwin, H.J. 1980. "Out-of-the-Body Down Under: Some Cognitive Characteristics of Australian Students Reporting OBEs." *Journal of the Society for Psychical Research* 50(785):448–59.
James, W. 1961. *The Varieties of Religious Experience*. New York: Crowell-Collier.

Kohr, R.L. 1980. "A Survey of Psi Experiences Among Members of a Special Population." *Journal of the American Society for Psychical Research* 74:395–411.

Maslow, A.H. (1970). *Religious Values and Peak Experiences*. New York: The Viking Press.

Mauskopf, S.H., and M.R. McVaugh. 1980. *The Elusive Science: Origins of Experimental Psychical Research*. Baltimore: The John Hopkins University Press.

Monroe, R.A. 1977. *Journeys Out-of-the-Body*. 2nd ed. New York: Anchor Books.

Muldoon, S., and H. Carrington. 1969. *The Phenomena of Astral Projection*. New York: Samuel Weiser, Inc. (first published, 1951).

Murdock, G.P. 1963. *Outline of World Cultures*. 3rd revised edition, New Haven: Human Relations Area Files, Inc.

Myers, F.W.H. 1903. *Human Personality and its Survival of Bodily Death*. London: Longmans.

Myers, S., H. Austrin, J. Grisso, and R. Nickeson. 1983. "Personality Characteristics as Related to Out-of-Body Experience." *Journal of Parapsychology* 47:131–44.

Osis, K. 1979. "Insiders' Views of the OBE: A Questionnaire Survey." *Research in Parapsychology—1978*. Metuchen, NJ: The Scarecrow Press, pp. 50–53.

———. 1973. "Perspectives for Out-of-Body Research." *Research in Parapsychology—1972*. Metuchen, NJ: Scarecrow Press.

Palmer, J. 1979. "A Community Mail Survey of Psychic Experiences." *Journal of the American Society for Psychical Research* 73(3):221–51.

Palmer, J., and C. Vassar. 1974. "ESP and Out-of-the-Body Experiences: An Exploratory Study." *Journal of the American Society for Psychical Research* 68:257–77.

Rogo, D.S. 1984. "Researching the Out-of-the-Body Experience: The State of the Art." *Anabiosis* 4:21–49.

———. 1975. "Some Musical Out-of-the-Body Experiences: A Brief Analysis." *Parapsychology Review*, Jan.-Feb., pp. 19–20.

Shiels, D. 1978. "A Cross-cultural Study of Beliefs in Out-of-the-Body Experiences, Waking and Sleeping." *Journal of the Society for Psychical Research* 49(775):697–741.

Smith, P., and H. Irwin. 1981. "Out-of-Body Experiences, Needs and the Experimental Approach: A Laboratory Study." *Parapsychology Review* 12(3):1–4.

Tart, C.T. 1972. "States of Consciousness and State Specific Sciences." *Science* 176:1203–10.

———. 1971. *On Being Stoned: A Psychological Study of Marijuana Intoxication*. Palo Alto: Science and Behavior Books.

Twemlow, S.W., G.O. Gabbard, and F.C. Jones. 1982. "The Out-of-Body Experience: A Phenomenological Typology Based on Questionnaire Responses." *American Journal of Psychiatry* 139(4):450–55.

Whiteman, J.H.M. 1956. "The Process of Separation and Return in Experiences Fully 'Out of the Body'." *Proceedings of the Society for Psychical Research* 50(185):240–74.

Yram (pseudonym). 1965. *Practical Astral Projection*. New York: Samuel Weiser, Inc.

CHAPTER TWO

American Psychiatric Association. 1980. *Diagnostic and Statistical Manual of Mental Disorders*. 3rd ed. Washington, DC: American Psychiatric Association.

Blackmore, S.J. 1984. "A Postal Survey of OBE's and Other Experiences." *Journal of the Society for Psychical Research* 52(796):225–44.

Caine, T.M. 1972. "Personality and Illness." In *Psychological Assessment of Mental and Physical Handicaps*, edited by P. Mittler. New York: Methuen.

Dickstein, L.S. 1972. "Death Concern: Measurements and Correlates." *Psychological Reports* 30:563–71.

Ellsworth, R.B. 1981. "Profile of Adaptation to Life." Consulting Psychology Press. P.O. Box 16636; Palo Alto, CA 94306.

Eysenck, S.B.G., and H.J. Eysenck. 1968. "The Measurement of Psychoticism: A Study of Factor Stability and Reliability." *British Journal Social and Clinical Psychology* 7:286–94.

Giovetti, P. 1983. "Out-of-Body Experiences: An Italian Survey." *Theta* 11(3): 63–66.

Green, C.E. 1968. *Out-of-the-Body Experiences*. London: Hamish Hamilton.

———. 1967. "Ecsomatic Experiences and Related Phenomena." *Journal of the Society for Psychical Research* 44(733):111–30.

Hood, R.W., J.R. Hall, P.J. Watson, and M. Biderman. 1979. "Personality Correlates of the Report of Mystical Experience." *Psychological Reports* 44: 804–6.

Irwin, H.J. 1981. "The Psychological Function of Out-of-Body Experiences. So Who Needs the Out-of-Body Experience?" *Journal of Nervous Mental Diseases* 169(4):244–48.

———. 1980. "Out-of-the-Body Down Under: Some Cognitive Characteristics of Australian Students Reporting OBEs." *Journal of the Society for Psychical Research* 50(785):448–59.

Jones, F.C., G.O. Gabbard, and S.W. Twemlow. 1984. "Psychological and Demographic Characteristics of Persons Reporting Out-of-Body Experiences." *Hillside Journal of Clinical Psychiatry*. 6(1):105-115.

Kennedy, R.B. 1976. "Self-induced Depersonalization Syndrome." *American Journal of Psychiatry* 133:1326–28.

Maliszewski, M., S.W. Twemlow, D.P. Brown, and J.M. Engler. 1981. "A Phenomenological Typology of Intensive Meditation: A Suggested Methodology Using the Questionnaire Approach." *ReVision* 4(2):3–27.

Myers, S., H. Austrin, J. Grisso, and R. Nickeson. 1983. "Personality Characteristics as Related to the Out-of-Body Experience." *Journal of Parapsychology* 47:131–44.

Osis, K. 1979. "Insider's View of the OBE: A Questionnaire Survey." *Research in Parapsychology—1978*. Metuchen, NJ: The Scarecrow Press, pp. 50–53.

Palmer, J. 1979. "A Community Mail Survey of Psychic Experiences." *Journal of the American Society for Psychical Research* 73(3):221–51.

Palmer, J., and R. Lieberman. 1976. "E.S.P. and Out-of-Body Experiences: A Further Study." *Research in Parapsychology*, pp. 102–6.

"Profile of Moods Scale: Educational and Industrial Testing Service." 1971. San Diego, CA 92107.

Quay, H.C. 1965. "Psychopathic Personality as Pathological Stimulation Seeking." *American Journal of Psychiatry* 122:180-83.

Tellegen, A., and G. Atkinson. 1974. "Openness to Absorbing and Self-Altering Experiences ('Absorption'): A Trait Related to Hypnotic Susceptibility." *Journal of Abnormal Psychology* 53:368–77.

Twemlow, S.W., and G.O. Gabbard. In press. "The Influence of Demographic/ Psychological Factors and Pre-existing Conditions on the Near-Death Experience." *Omega*.

Walsh, R. 1980. "The Consciousness Disciplines and the Behavioral Sciences: Questions of Comparison and Assessment." *American Journal of Psychiatry* 137:663–73.

Wilson, S., and T. Barber. 1982. "The Fantasy-Prone Personality: Implications for Understanding Imagery, Hypnosis and Parapsychological Phenomena." In *Imagery: Current Theory, Research and Application*, edited by A.A. Sheikh. New York: John Wiley.

CHAPTER THREE

Acker, B. 1954. "Depersonalization: I. Aetiology and Phenomenology." *Journal of Mental Science* 100:838–53.

Ambrosino, S. 1973. "Phobic Anxiety—Depersonalization Syndrome." *New York State Journal of Medicine* 73:419–25.

American Psychiatric Association. 1980. *Diagnostic and Statistical Manual of Mental Disorders*. 3rd ed. Washington, DC: American Psychiatric Association.

Arlow, J. 1966. "Depersonalization and Derealization." In *Psychoanalysis— A General Psychology: Essays in Honor of Heinz Hartmann*, edited by R. Loewenstein et al. New York: International Universities Press.

Bergler, E., and Eidelberg, L. 1935. "Der Mechanismus Der Depersonalisation." *Int. Z. Psychoanal.* 21:258–85.

Blank, H. 1954. "Depression, Hypomania, and Depersonalization." *Psychoanalytic Quarterly* 23:20–37.

Federn, P. 1952. *Ego Psychology and the Psychoses*. New York: Basic Books.

Fenichel, O. 1945. *The Psychoanalytic Theory of Neurosis*. New York: Norton.

Fisher, S., and Seidner, R. 1963. "Body Experiences of Schizophrenic, Neurotic, and Normal Women." *Journal of Nervous and Mental Disease* 137:252–57.

Freud, S. 1936. "A Disturbance of Memory on the Acropolis." *S.E.* 22.

———. 1918. "From the History of an Infantile Neurosis." *S.E.* 17.

Gabbard, G.O. 1983. "Further Contributions to the Understanding of Stage Fright: Narcissistic Issues." *Journal of the American Psychoanalytic Association* 31:324–41.

———. 1979. "Stage Fright." *International Journal of Psychoanalysis* 60:383–92.

Gabbard, G.O., S.W. Twemlow, and F.C. Jones. 1982. "Differential Diagnosis of Altered Mind/Body Perception." *Psychiatry* 45:361–69.

Jacobson, E. 1959. "Depersonalization." *Journal of the American Psychoanalytic Association* 7:581–610.

Kennedy, R. 1976. "Self-Induced Depersonalization Syndrome." *American Journal of Psychiatry* 133:1326–28.

Kohut, H. 1977. *The Restoration of the Self*. New York: International Universities Press.

Myers, W. 1976. "Imaginary Companions, Fantasy Twins, Mirror Dreams, and Depersonalization." *The Psychoanalytic Quarterly* 45:503–24.

Nemiah, J. 1980. "Depersonalization Disorder." In *Comprehensive Textbook of Psychiatry*, Vol. 3, edited by A. Freedman, H. Kaplan, and B. Sadock. Baltimore: Williams and Wilkins.

Noyes, R., and R. Kletti. 1976. "Depersonalization in the Face of Life-Threatening Danger: A Description." *Psychiatry* 39:19–27.

Noyes, R., P. Hoenk, S. Kuperman, and D. Slymen. 1977. "Depersonalization in Accident Victims and Psychiatric Patients." *Journal of Nervous and Mental Disease* 164:401–7.

Nunberg, H. 1932. *Principles of Psychoanalysis: Their Application to the Neuroses*. New York: International Universities Press, 1955.

Roberts, W. 1960. "Normal and Abnormal Depersonalization." *Journal of Mental Science* 106:478–93.

Rosenfeld, H. 1947. "Analysis of a Schizophrenic State with Depersonaliza-

tion." In *Psychotic States: A Psychoanalytical Approach*. New York: International Universities Press, 1966.
Sabom, M. 1982. *Recollections of Death*. New York: Harper and Row.
Sarlin, C. 1962. "Depersonalization and Derealization." *Journal of the American Psychoanalytic Association* 10:784–804.
Schilder, P. 1935. *The Image and Appearance of the Human Body*. London: Routledge and Kegan Paul.
Selinsky, H. 1968. "Depersonalization and Derealization: Review of Present Day Concepts." *Journal of Hillside Hospital* 17:306–16.
Stamm, J. 1962. "Altered Ego States Allied to Depersonalization." *Journal of the American Psychoanalytic Association* 10:762–83.
Stolorow, R. 1979. "Defensive and Arrested Developmental Aspects of Death Anxiety, Hypochondriasis and Depersonalization." *International Journal of Psycho-Analysis* 60:201–13.
Tucker, G., M. Harrow, and D. Quinlan. 1973. "Depersonalization, Dysphoria, and Thought Disturbance." *American Journal of Psychiatry* 130:702–6.
Waelder, R. 1930. "The Principle of Multiple Function: Observations on Overdetermination." In *Psychoanalysis: Observation, Theory, and Application. Selected papers of Robert Waelder*, edited by S. Guttman. New York: International Universities Press, 1976.

CHAPTER FOUR

Alonso-Fernandez, F. 1976. *Fundamentos de la Psiquiatria Actual*, vol. 1, 3rd ed. Madrid: Paz Montalvo.
Bion, W. 1957. "Differentiation of the Psychotic From the Nonpsychotic Personality." In *Second Thoughts*. London: William Heinemann, 1967.
Bogaert, L. 1934. "Sur La Pathologie de L'image de Soi." *Annales Medico-Psychologiques* 92:744–59.
Coleman, S. 1934. "The Phantom Double: Its Psychological Significance." *British Journal of Medical Psychology* 14:254–73.
Damas Mora, J., F. Jenner, and S. Eacott. 1980. "On Heautoscopy or the Phenomenon of the Double: Case Presentation and Review of the Literature." *British Journal of Medical Psychology* 53:75–83.
Dewhurst, K. 1954. "Autoscopic Hallucinations." *Irish Journal of Medical Science* 1:263–67.
Dewhurst, K., and J. Pearson. 1955. "Visual Hallucinations of the Self in Organic Disease." *Journal of Neurology, Neurosurgery, and Psychiatry* 18:53–57.
Faguet, R. 1979. "With the Eyes of the Mind: Autoscopic Phenomena in the Hospital Setting." *General Hospital Psychiatry* 1:311–14.
Freud, S. 1919. "The 'Uncanny'." *S. E.* 17:217–56.

Gazzaniga, M., and J. Ledoux. 1978. *The Integrated Mind*. New York: Plenum Press.
Green, C. 1968. *Out-of-Body Experiences*. London: Hamish Hamilton.
Grotstein, J. 1983. "Autoscopy: The Experience of One's Self as a Double." *The Hillside Journal of Clinical Psychiatry* 5:259–304.
———. 1982. "Autoscopic Phenomena." In *Extraordinary Disorders of Human Behavior*, edited by C. Friedmann and R. Faguet. New York: Plenum Press.
Hamilton, J. 1979. "The Doppelgänger Effect in the Relationship Between Joseph Conrad and Bertrand Russell." *International Review of Psycho-Analysis* 6:175–81.
———. 1975. "The Significance of Depersonalization in the Life and Writings of Joseph Conrad." *Psychoanalytic Quarterly* 44:612–30.
Katan, M. 1954. "The Importance of the Non-psychotic Part of the Personality in Schizophrenia." *International Journal of Psycho-Analysis* 35:119–28.
Kohut, H. 1971. *The Analysis of the Self*. New York: International Universities Press.
Lhermitte, J. 1951. "Visual Hallucination of the Self." *British Medical Journal* 1:431–34.
———. 1948. "De L'image Corporelle et de ses Deformations Pathologiques." *Folia Psychiatrique Neurologique et Neurochirurgique (Neerl)* 51:374–79.
Lukianowicz, N. 1958. "Autoscopic Phenomena." *AMA Archives of Neurology and Psychiatry* 80:199–220.
Lunn, V. 1970. "Autoscopic Phenomena." *Acta Psychiatrica Scandinavica* 46 Supplement 219:118–25.
Menninger-Lerchenthal, E. 1935. "Das Truggebilde der eigenen Gestalt (Heautoscopie Doppelgänger)." *Abhandlungen aus der Neurologic* 74:1.
Ostow, N. 1960. "The Metapsychology of Autoscopic Phenomena." *International Journal of Psycho-Analysis* 41:619–25.
Rank, O. 1971. *The Double—A Psychoanalytic Study*. New York: New American Library.
Sabom, N. 1982. *Recollections of Death*. New York: Harper and Row.
Sollier, P. 1903. *Les Phenomenes d'Autoscopie*. Paris: F. Alcan.
Tausk, V. 1919. "On The Origin of the 'Influencing Machine' in Schizophrenia." In *Psychoanalytic Reader*, edited by R. Fleiss. New York: International Universities Press, 1948, pp. 52–85.
Wigan, A. 1844. *The Duality of the Mind: A New View of Insanity*. London: Longman, Brown, Green and Longman.

CHAPTER FIVE

Angyal, A. 1935. "The Perceptual Basis of Somatic Delusions in a Case of Schizophrenia." *Archives of Neurology and Psychiatry* 34:270.

Blatt, S., and C. Wild. 1976. *Schizophrenia: A Developmental Approach*. New York: Academic Press.
Burton, A., and J. Adkins. 1961. "Perceived Size of Self-image Body Parts in Schizophrenia." *Archives of General Psychiatry* 5:39.
Cardone, S., and R. Olson. 1969. "Chlorpromazine and Body Image." *Archives of General Psychiatry* 20:576–82.
Chapman, L., J. Chapman, and N. Raulin. 1978. "Body-Image Aberration in Schizophrenia." *Journal of Abnormal Psychology* 87:399–407.
Cleveland, S. 1960. "Judgments of Body Size in a Schizophrenic and a Control Group." *Psychological Reports* 7:304.
Darby, J. 1970. "Alteration of Some Body Image Indexes in Schizophrenics." *Journal of Consulting and Clinical Psychology* 35:116–21.
Dillon, D. 1962. "Measurement of Perceived Body Size." *Perceptual and Motor Skills* 14:191–96.
Federn, P. 1952. *Ego Psychology and the Psychoses*. New York: Basic Books.
Fisher, S. 1966. "Body Image in Neurotic and Schizophrenic Patients." *Archives of General Psychiatry* 17:90–101.
Fisher, S., and S. Cleveland. 1968. *Body Image and Personality*, 2nd ed. New York: Dover Publications.
Fisher, S., and R. Seidner. 1963. "Body Experiences of Schizophrenic, Neurotic, and Normal Women." *Journal of Nervous and Mental Disease* 137:252–57.
Freedman, N. et al. 1965. "Communication of Body Complaints and Paranoid Symptoms Change Under Conditions of Phenothiazine Treatment." *Journal of Personality and Social Psychology* 1:310–18.
Freeman, T., J. Cameron, and A. McGhie. 1958. *Chronic Schizophrenia*. New York: International Universities Press.
Freud, S. 1923. "The Ego and The Id." *S. E.*, 19.
Goertzel, V., P. May, J. Salkin, and T. Schoop. 1965. "Body-Ego Technique: An Approach to the Schizophrenic Patient." *Journal of Nervous and Mental Disease* 141:53–60.
Grand, S. 1982. "The Body and Its Boundaries: A Psychoanalytic View of Cognitive Process Disturbances in Schizophrenia." *International Review of Psycho-Analysis* 9:327–42.
Holtzman, W., J. Thorpe, J. Swartz, and E. Herron. 1961. *Ink-Blot Perception and Personality*. Austin: University of Texas Press.
Jenkins, S., and A. Sambroski. 1964. "Symptom Specificity of Anti-Psychotic Drugs." *Journal of the Michigan Medical Society* 63:187–93.
Kokonis, N. 1972. "Body Image Disturbance in Schizophrenia: A Study of Arms and Feet." *Journal of Personality Assessment* 36:573–75.
Lancaster, N. 1954. "Body Image Disturbances." *Lancet* 1:81.
Lidz, T., S. Fleck, and A. Corenlison. 1965. *Schizophrenia and the Family*. New York: International Universities Press.

Lukianowicz, N. 1967. "'Body Image' Disturbances in Psychiatric Disorders." *British Journal of Psychiatry* 113:31–47.

Mahler, N. 1952. "On Child Psychosis and Schizophrenia: Autistic and Symbiotic Infantile Psychoses." *Psychoanalytic Study of the Child* 7:286–305.

Mantegazza, P. 1859. "On the Hygienic and Medicinal Virtues of Coca." In *The Coca Leaf and Cocaine Papers*, edited by G. Andrews and D. Solomon. New York: Harcourt Brace Jovanovich, 1975.

Papson, D., and R. Hamersma. 1974. "Perceptions of Schizophrenics versus Normals Using Parental Figures and Subject's Size." *Perceptual and Motor Skills* 38:711–16.

Quinlan, D., and N. Harrow. 1974. "Boundary Disturbances in Schizophrenia." *Journal of Abnormal Psychology* 83:533–41.

Schilder, P. 1935. *The Image and Appearance of the Human Body*. London: Kegan Paul, Trench, Trubner and Company.

Shukla, T. 1972. "Perception of Penetration of Body-Image-Boundary in Schizophrenia." *Psychologia* 15:240–42.

Tausk, V. 1919. "On the Origin of the Influencing Machine in Schizophrenia." *Psychoanalytic Quarterly* 2:519–56.

Traub, A., R. Olson, J. Orbach, and S. Cardone. 1967. "Psycho-Physical Studies of Body-Image: III. Initial Studies of Disturbances in a Chronic Schizophrenic Group." *Archives of General Psychiatry* 17:664–70.

Weckowicz, T., and R. Sommer. 1960. "Body Image and Self-Concept in Schizophrenia, An Experimental Study." *Journal of Mental Science* 106:17–39.

CHAPTER SIX

Antrobus, J.S. 1968. "Information Theory and Stimulus Independent Thought." *British Journal of Psychology* 59:423–30.

Antrobus, J.S., R. Coleman, and J.L. Singer. 1967. "Signal Detection Performance by Subjects Differing in Predisposition to Daydreaming." *Journal of Consulting Psychology* 31:487–91.

Arkin, A.M., J.S. Antrobus, and S.J. Ellman, editors. 1978. *The Mind in Sleep: Psychology and Psychophysiology*. New York: John Wiley and Sons.

Aserinsky, E., and N. Kleitman. 1953. "Regularly Occurring Periods of Eye Motility and Concomitant Phenomena During Sleep." *Science* 118:273–74.

Beit-Hallahmi, B. 1972. "Developing the Prison Fantasy Questionnaire (P.F.Q.)." *Journal of Clinical Psychology* 28:552–54.

Blackmore, S.J. 1982. "Out-of-Body Experiences, Lucid Dreams, and Imagery: Two Surveys." *Journal of the American Society for Psychical Research* 76(4):301–17.

Bliss, E.L., and L.D. Clark. 1962. "Visual Hallucinations." In *Hallucinations*, edited by L.J. West. New York: Grune & Stratton.

Brown, D.P. 1977. "Levels of Concentrative Meditation." *International Journal of Clinical and Experimental Hypnosis* 25(4):9236–73.

Carr, D. 1982. "Pathophysiology of Stress-Induced Limbic Lobe Dysfunction: A Hypothesis for NDEs." *Anabiosis* 2(1):75–89.

Castaneda, C. 1972. *Journey to Ixtlan*. New York: Simon and Schuster.

Crookall, R. 1965. *Intimations of Immortality*. London: James Clarke.

Faraday, A. 1974. *The Dream Game*. New York: Harper and Row.

———. 1972. *Dream Power*. New York: Coward, McCann, and Geoghegan.

Federn, P. 1952. *Ego Psychology and the Psychoses*. New York: Basic Books.

Foulkes, D. 1962. "Dream Reports from Different Stages of Sleep." *Journal of Abnormal and Social Psychology* 65:14–25.

Foulkes, D., and Vogel, G. 1966. "Mental Activity at Sleep Onset." *Journal of Abnormal Psychology* 70(4):231–43.

Fox, O. (pseudonym). 1962. *Astral Projection: A Record of Out-of-Body Experiences*. Secaucus, NJ: University Books. (originally published in 1939).

Freedman, A.M., H.L. Kaplan, and B.J. Sadock. 1975. *Comprehensive Textbook of Psychiatry*, vol. 1, 2nd ed. Baltimore: Williams & Wilkins.

Freedman, S.J., and P.A. Marks. 1965. "Visual Imagery Produced by Rhythmic Photic Stimulation; Personality Correlates and Phenomenology." *British Journal Psychology* 56:95–112.

Freud, S. 1908. *Creative Writers and Daydreaming*. S.E. 9.

———. 1900. *The Interpretation of Dreams*. S.E. 4 and 5.

Gackenbach, J.I. 1979. "A Personality and Cognitive Style Analysis of Lucid Dreaming." *Dissertation Abstracts International* 39, No. 7.

Giambra, L.M. 1982. "Daydreaming: A Black-White Comparison for 17–34 Year Olds." *Journal of Personality and Social Psychology* 42(6):1146–56.

———. 1974. "Daydreaming Across the Lifespan: Late Adolescent to Senior Citizen." *Aging and Human Development* 5:116–35.

Gordon, R. 1962. "Stereotypy of Imagery and Belief as an Ego Defense." *British Journal of Psychology* 24:1–96.

———. 1949. "An Investigation into Some of the Factors that Favor the Formation of Sterotyped Images." *British Journal of Psychology* 39:156–67.

Green, C. 1968a. "Out-of-the-Body Experiences." London: Hamish Hamilton.

———. 1968b. "Lucid Dreams." Oxford: Volume 1 of Proceedings of the Institute of Psychophysical Research.

———. 1966. "Spontaneous 'Paranormal' Experiences in Relation to Sex and

Academic Background." *Journal of the Society for Psychical Research* 43:357–63.

Greyson, B. 1983. "Near-Death Experiences and Personal Values." *American Journal of Psychiatry* 140(5):618–20.

Grotstein, J.S. In press. "A Proposed Revision of the Psychoanalytic Concept of Primitive Mental States. Part II. The Borderline Syndrome." *Contemporary Psychoanalysis*.

Hariton, E.B., and J.L. Singer. 1974. "Womens' Fantasies During Sexual Intercourse: Normative and Theoretical Implications." *Journal of Consulting and Clinical Psychology* 42:313–22.

Horowitz, M.J. 1970. *Image Formation and Cognition*. New York: Appleton-Century-Crofts.

Irwin, H.J. 1980. "Out-of-the-Body Down Under: Some Cognitive Characteristics of Australian Students Reporting OBEs." *Journal of the Society for Psychical Research* 50(785):448–59.

Isaacs, D. 1975. "Cognitive Styles in Daydreaming." Doctoral dissertation. New York: City University. Reported in Singer, J.L. "Navigating the Stream of Consciousness." *American Psychologist* 30(7):727–38.

Isakower, O. 1938. "A Contribution to the Pathophysiology of Phenomena Associated with Falling Asleep." *International Journal of Psychoanalysis* 19:331–45.

James, W. 1961. *The Varieties of Religious Experience*. New York: Collier Books.

———. 1950. (Originally published in 1890.) *The Principles of Psychology*, vol. 1. New York: Dover.

Jones, F.C., G.O. Gabbard, and S.W. Twemlow. 1984. "Psychological and Demographic Characteristics of Persons Reporting Out-of-Body Experiences." *Hillside Journal of Clinical Psychiatry* 6(1):105-115.

Kennedy, R.B., Jr. 1976. "Self-Induced Depersonalization Syndrome." *American Journal of Psychiatry* 133:1326–28.

Klinger, E. 1978-79. "Dimensions of Thought and Imagery in Normal Waking States." *Journal Altered States of Consciousness* 4(2):97–112.

Kohr, R.L. 1980. "A Survey of Psi Experiences Among Members of a Special Population." *Journal of the American Society for Psychical Research* 74:395–411.

Kramer, M., editor. 1969. *Dream Psychology and the New Biology of Dreaming*. Springfield, Ill: Charles C. Thomas.

LaBerge, S.P. 1981. "Lucid Dreaming: Directing the Action as it Happens." *Psychology Today* 15(1):48–57.

LaBerge, S.P., L.E. Nagel, W.C. Dement, and U.P. Zarcone. 1981. "Lucid Dreaming Verified by Volitional Communication During REM Sleep." *Perceptual and Motor Skills* 52(3):727–32.

LaBerge, S.P. 1980. "Lucid Dreaming and a Learnable Skill: A Case Study." *Perceptual and Motor Skills* 51(3):1039–42.
Leaning, F.E. 1926. "An Introductory Study of Hypnagogic Phenomena." *Proceedings Society for Psychical Research* 35:289–409.
Maury, L.F.A. 1861. "Le Sommeil et les Reves, Paris." Quoted in Richardson, A.L. 1969. *Mental Imagery*. New York: Springer.
McKellar, P. 1972. *Imagery from the Standpoint of Introspection, In the Function and Nature of Imagery*, edited by P.W. Sheehan, pp. 35-61. New York: Academic Press.
———. 1957. *Imagination and Thinking*. New York: Basic Books.
McKellar, P., and L. Simpson. 1954. "Between Wakefulness and Sleep: Hypnagogic Imagery." *British Journal of Psychology* 45:266–76.
Monroe, R.A. 1977. *Journeys Out of the Body*. New York: Anchor Books.
Morris, R.L, S.B. Harary, J. Janis, J. Hartwell, and W.G. Ross. 1978. "Studies of Communication During Out-of-Body Experiences." *Journal of the American Society for Psychical Research* 72:1–21.
Muldoon, S., and H. Carrington. 1977. *The Projection of the Astral Body*. New York: Samuel Weiser. (originally published in 1929.)
Myers, F.W.H. 1903. *Human Personality and Its Survival of Bodily Death*. London: Longmans Green.
Palmer, J. 1979. "A Community Mail Survey of Psychic Experiences." *Journal of the American Society for Psychical Research* 73:221–51.
Pinard, W.J. 1957. "Spontaneous Imagery: Its Nature, Therapeutic Value and Effect on Personality Structure." *Boston University Graduate Journal* 5:150–53.
Pivik, T., and D. Foulkes. 1968. "NREM Mentation: Relation to Personality, Orientation Time, and Time of Night." *Journal of Consulting and Clinical Psychology* 37:144–51.
Richardson, A. 1969. *Mental Imagery*. New York: Springer.
Richard, J.T., A. Mauromatic, T. Mindel, and A.C. Owens. 1981. "Individual Differences in Hypnagogic and Hypnopompic Imagery." *Journal of Mental Imagery* 5(2):91–96.
Salley, R.D. 1982. "REM Sleep Phenomena During Out-of-Body Experiences." *Journal of the American Society for Psychical Research* 76:157–65.
Shapiro, D. 1965. *Neurotic Styles*. New York: Basic Books.
Sharpe, E.F. 1961. *Dream Analysis*. London: The Hogarth Press.
Shiels, D. 1978. "A Cross-Cultural Study of Beliefs in Out-of-the-Body Experiences, Waking and Sleeping." *Journal of the Society for Psychical Research* 49(775):697–741.
Schlauch, R. 1979. "Hypnopompic Hallucinations and Treatment with Imipramine." *American Journal of Psychiatry* 136(2):219–20.
Siegel, R.K. 1980. "The Psychology of Life After Death." *American Psychologist* 35:911–31.

Singer, J.L. 1975a. "Navigating the Stream of Consciousness: Research in Daydreaming and Related Inner Experiences." *American Psychologist* 30(7): 727–38.
———. 1975b. *The Inner World of Daydreaming*. New York: Harper and Row.
Singer, J.L., and K.S. Pope. 1980. "Daydreaming and Imagery Skills as Predisposing Capacities for Self-Hypnosis." *The International Journal of Clinical and Experimental Hypnosis* 29(3): 271–81.
Snyder, F. 1969. *The Physiology of Dreaming in Dream Psychology and the New Biology of Dreaming*, edited by M. Kramer. Springfield, Ill: Charles C. Thomas.
Sparrow, G.S. 1975. "Lucid Dreaming as an Evolutionary Process." *The A.R.E. Journal* 10(3):1–19.
Starker, S., and J.L. Singer. 1975. "Daydreaming and Symptom Patterns of Psychiatric Patients: A Factor Analytic Study." *Journal of Abnormal Psychology* 84(5):567–70.
Tart, C.T. 1968. "A Psychophysiological Study of Out-of-Body Experiences in a Selected Subject." *Journal of the American Society for Psychical Research* 62:3–27.
Tellegen, A., and G. Atkinson. 1974. "Openness to Absorbing and Self-Altering Experiences ('Absorption'): A Trait Related to Hypnotic Susceptibility." *Journal of Abnormal Psychology* 53:368–77.
Thale, T., G. Westcott, and K. Salomon. 1950. "Hallucinations and Imagery Induced by Mescaline." *American Journal of Psychiatry* 106:686–91.
Twemlow, S.W. 1977. "Epilogue: Personality File." In *Journeys Out-of-the-Body*, by R.A. Monroe, pp. 275–80. New York: Anchor Books.
Twemlow, S.W., G.O. Gabbard, and F.C. Jones. 1982. "The Out-of-Body Experience: A Phenomenological Typology Based on Questionnaire Responses." *American Journal of Psychiatry* 139(4):450–55.
Van Eeden, F. 1913. (Reprinted in C.T. Tart, 1969. *Altered States of Consciousness*. New York: John Wiley & Sons.) *A Study of Dreams*. *Proceedings of the Society for Psychical Research* 26:431–61.
Vernon, J.A. 1963. *Inside the Black Room*. New York: Clarkson N. Potter.
Whiteman, J.H.M. 1956. "The Process of Separation and Return in Experiences Fully 'Out-of-Body'." *Proceedings of the Society for Psychical Research* 50:240–74.
Zorick, F.J., P.J. Salis, T. Roth, and M. Kramer. 1979. "Narcolepsy and Automatic Behavior: A Case Report." *Journal of Clinical Psychiatry* 40(4): 194–97.

CHAPTER SEVEN

Becker, C.B. 1982. "The Failure of Saganomics: Why Birth Models Cannot Explain Near-Death Phenomena." *Anabiosis* 2:102–9.

Carr, D. 1982. "Pathophysiology of Stress-Induced Limbic Lobe Dysfunction: A Hypothesis for NDEs." *Anabiosis* 2:75-89.

Ehrenwald, J. 1974. "Out-of-the-Body Experiences and the Denial of Death." *Journal of Nervous and Mental Disease* 159:227-33.

Gabbard, G.O., and S.W. Twemlow. 1981. "Explanatory Hypotheses for Near-Death Experiences." *ReVision* 4:68-71.

Gabbard, G.O., S.W. Twemlow, and F.C. Jones. 1981. "Do 'Near-Death Experiences' Occur Only Near Death?" *The Journal of Nervous and Mental Disease* 169:374-77.

Gallup, G. with W. Porter. 1982. *Adventures in Immortality: A Look Beyond the Threshold of Death.* New York: McGraw Hill.

Greyson, B. 1983. "The Psychodynamics of Near-Death Experiences." *The Journal of Nervous and Mental Disease* 171:376-81.

———. 1981a. "Toward a Psychological Explanation of Near-Death Experiences: A Response to Dr. Grosso's Paper." *Anabiosis* 1:88-103.

———. 1981b. "Near-Death Experiences and Attempted Suicide." *Suicide and Life Threatening Behavior* 11:10-16.

Greyson, B., and I. Stevenson. 1980. "The Phenomenology of Near-Death Experiences." *American Journal of Psychiatry* 137:1193-96.

Grof, S. 1975. *Realms of the Human Unconscious.* New York: Viking.

Grosso, M. 1981. "Toward an Explanation of Near-Death Phenomena." *Anabiosis* 1:3-26.

McHarg, J.F. 1978. Review of *At the Hour of Death*, by Osis and Haraldsson. *Journal of the Society for Psychical Research* 49:885-87.

Moody, R.A., Jr. 1975. *Life After Life.* Atlanta: Mockingbird Books.

Noyes, R. 1981. "The Subjective Response to Life Threatening Danger." Presented at the Annual Meeting of the American Psychiatric Association in New Orleans, Louisiana.

———. 1972. "The Experience of Dying." *Psychiatry* 35:174-84.

Noyes, R., and R. Kletti. 1976a. "Depersonalization in the Face of Life Threatening Danger: A Description." *Psychiatry* 39:19-27.

———. 1976b. "Depersonalization in the Face of Life Threatening Danger: An Interpretation." *Omega* 7:103-14.

———. 1977a. "Depersonalization in Response to Life Threatening Danger." *Comprehensive Psychiatry* 18:375-84.

———. 1977b. "Panoramic Memory: A Response to the Threat of Death." *Omega* 8:181-94.

Osis, K., and E. Haraldsson. 1977. *At the Hour of Death.* New York: Avon Books.

Ring, K. 1982. Review of *Adventures in Immortality: A Look Beyond the Threshold* by G. Gallup with W. Porter. *Anabiosis* 2:160-65.

———. 1980. *Life at Death: A Scientific Investigation of the Near-Death Experience.* New York: Coward, McCann, and Geoghegan.

Rodin, E.A. 1980. "The Reality of Death Experiences." *The Journal of Nervous and Mental Disease* 168:259–63.
Sabom, M. 1982. *Recollections of Death*. New York: Harper and Row.
Sabom, M., and S. Kreutziger. 1977. "Near-Death Experiences." *New England Journal of Medicine* 297:1071.
Sagan, C. 1979. *Broca's Brain*. New York: Random House.
Siegel, R.K. 1980. "The Psychology of Life After Death." *American Psychologist* 35:911–31.
Twemlow, S.W., G.O. Gabbard, and L. Coyne. 1982. "A Multivariate Method for the Classification of Pre-Existing Near-Death Conditions." *Anabiosis* 2:139–39.

CHAPTER EIGHT

Becker, C. 1981. "The Centrality of Near-Death Experience in Chinese Pure Land Buddhism." *Anabiosis* 1:154–71.
Caine, R. 1972. "Personality and Illness." In *Psychological Assessment of Mental and Physical Handicaps*, edited by P. Mittler. New York: Metheun.
Davidson, R., D. Goleman, and G. Schwartz. 1976. "Attentional and Affective Concomitants of Meditation: A Cross-Sectional Study." *Journal of Abnormal Psychology* 85:235–38.
Dickstein, L. 1972. "Death Concern: Measurement and Correlates." *Psychological Reports* 30:563–71.
Dobson, M., A. Tattersifle, and M. Adler. 1971. "Attitudes and Long-Term Adjustment of Patients Surviving Cardiac Arrest." *British Medical Journal* 3:207–12.
Druss, R., and D. Kornfield. 1967. "The Survivors of Cardiac Arrest: A Psychiatric Study." *Journal of the American Medical Association* 201:291–96.
Eysenck, S., and H. Eysenck. 1968. "The Measure of Psychoticism: A Study of Factor Stability and Reliability." *British Journal of Social and Clinical Psychology* 7:286–94.
Friedman, H., and J. Rubin. 1967. "On Some Invariant Criteria for Grouping Data." *Journal of the American Statistical Association* 62:1149–78.
Gabbard, G.O., S.W. Twemlow, and F.C. Jones. 1981. "Do 'Near-Death Experiences' Occur Only Near Death?" *Journal of Nervous and Mental Disease* 169:374–77.
Gallup, G., and W. Proctor. 1982. *Adventures in Immortality*. New York: McGraw-Hill.
Green, C. 1968. *Out-of-Body Experiences*. London: Hamish Hamilton.

Green, J., and P. Friedman. 1983. "Near-Death Experiences in a Southern California Population." *Anabiosis* 3:77–95.
Greyson, B., and I. Stevenson. 1980. "The Phenomenology of Near-Death Experiences." *American Journal of Psychiatry* 137:1193–96.
Grof, S., and J. Halifax. 1978. *The Human Encounter with Death.* New York: E. P. Dutton.
Irwin, H. 1980. "Out-of-the-Body Down Under: Some Cognitive Characteristics of Australian Students Reporting OBEs." *Journal of the Society for Psychical Research* 50:448–59.
Kohut, H. 1971. *The Analysis of the Self.* New York: International Universities Press.
Lindley, J., S. Bryan, and R. Conly. 1981. "Near-Death Experiences in a Pacific Northwest American Population: The Evergreen Study." *Anabiosis* 1:104–24.
Lundahl, C., and H. Widdison. 1983. "The Mormon Explanation of Near-Death Experiences." *Anabiosis* 3:97–106.
Noyes, R., and R. Kletti. 1977. "Panoramic Memory: A Response to the Threat of Death." *Omega* 8:181–94.
———. "Depersonalization in the Face of Life-Threatening Danger: A Description." *Psychiatry* 39:19–27.
Osis, K., and E. Haraldsson. 1977. *At the Hour of Death.* New York: Avon.
Palmer, J., and R. Lieberman. 1975. "The Influence of Psychological Set on ESP and Out-of-Body Experiences." *Journal of the American Society for Psychical Research* 69:193–213.
Ring, K. 1980. *Life At Death: A Scientific Investigation of the Near-Death Experience.* New York: Coward, McCann, and Geoghegan.
———. 1979. "Religiousness and Near-Death Experience: An Empirical Study." Presented at the American Psychological Association Annual Meeting, New York.
Rodin, E. 1980. "The Reality of Death Experiences." *Journal of Nervous and Mental Disease* 168:259–63.
Rosen, D. 1975. "Suicide Survivors: A Follow-up Study of Persons Who Survived Jumping from the Golden Gate and San Francisco-Oakland Bay Bridge." *Western Journal of Medicine* 122:289–94.
Sabom, M. 1980. "Commentary on 'The Reality of Death Experiences' by Ernst Rodin." *Journal of Nervous and Mental Disease* 168:266–67.
Schwarz, J. 1979. Personal Communication.
Siegel, R. 1980. "The Psychology of Life after Death." *American Psychologist* 25:911–31.
Smith, S. 1977. "The Golden Fantasy: A Regressive Reaction to Separation Anxiety." *International Journal of Psycho-Analysis* 58:311–24.
Stevenson, I., and B. Greyson. 1979. "Near-Death Experiences: Relevance to the Question of Survival After Death." *Journal of the American Medical Association* 242:265–67.

Tellegen, A., and G. Atkinson. 1974. "Openness to Absorbing and Self-Altering Experiences ('Absorption'): A Trait Related to Hypnotic Susceptibility." *Journal of Abnormal Psychology* 53:268–77.
Twemlow, S., G. Gabbard, and L. Coyne. 1982. "A Multivariate Method for the Classification of Pre-Existing Near-Death Conditions." *Anabiosis* 2:132–39.
Twemlow, S.W., and G.O. Gabbard. In press. "The Influence of Demographic/Psychological Factors and Pre-Existing Conditions on the Near-Death Experience." *Omega*.

CHAPTER NINE

Bush, N. 1984. "The Near-Death Experience in Children: Shades of the Prison-House Reopening." *Anabiosis* 3:177–93.
Khemka, K. 1983. Personal Communication.
Kohut, H. 1971. *The Analysis of the Self*. New York: International Universities Press.
Moody, R.A. 1975. *Life After Life*. Atlanta: Mockingbird Books.
Morse, M. 1983. "A Near Death Experience in a Seven-Year-Old Child." *American Journal of Diseases in Children* 137:959–61.
Sabom, M. 1982. *Recollections of Death*. New York: Harper and Row.
Sandler, J. 1960. "On the Concept of Superego." *Psychoanalytic Study of the Child* 15:128–62.
Schafer, R. 1960. "The Loving and Beloved Superego in Freud's Structural Theory." *Psychoanalytic Study of the Child* 15:163–88.
Smith, S. 1977. "The Golden Fantasy: A Regressive Reaction to Separation Anxiety." *International Journal of Psycho-Analysis* 58:311–24.
Ring, K. 1980. *Life At Death*. New York: Coward, McCann and Geoghegan.
Yalom, I. 1980. *Existential Psychotherapy*. New York: Basic Books.

CHAPTER TEN

Chattah, L. 1983. "Metapsychology: Its Cultural and Scientific Roots." Panel Report in *Journal of the American Psychoanalytic Association* 31:689–98.
Federn, P. 1952. *Ego Psychology and the Psychoses*. New York: Basic Books.
Freud, S. 1930. "Civilization and Its Discontents." *S.E.* 21.
———. 1923. "The Ego and the Id." *S.E.* 19.
———. 1900. "The Interpretation of Dreams." *S.E.* 4.
Gabbard, G. 1979. "Stage Fright." *International Journal of Psycho-Analysis* 60:383–92.

Grinberg, L., D. Sor, and E. Tabak de Bianchedi. 1977. *Introduction to the Work of Bion*. New York: Jason Aronson.

Hinsie, L., and R. Campbell. 1975. *Psychiatric Dictionary*. New York: Oxford University Press.

Kohut, H. 1971. *The Analysis of the Self*. New York: International Universities Press.

Mahler, M., and J. McDevitt. 1982. "Thoughts on the Emergence of the Sense of Self, with Particular Emphasis on the Body Self." *Journal of the American Psychoanalytic Association* 30:827–48.

Rinsley, D. 1962. "A Contribution to The Theory of Ego and Self." *Psychiatric Quarterly* 36:96–118.

Sartre, J. 1957. *The Transcendence of the Ego: An Existentialist Theory of Consciousness*, translated by F. Williams and B. Kirkpatrick. New York: Noonday Press.

Schilder, P. 1935. *The Image and Appearance of the Human Body*. London: Routledge and Kegan Paul.

CHAPTER ELEVEN

Becker, E. 1973. *The Denial of Death*. New York: The Free Press.

Blackmore, S. 1984. "Are Out-of-Body Experiences Evidence for Survival?" *Anabiosis* 3:137–53.

Brenner, C. 1955. *An Elementary Textbook of Psychoanalysis*. New York: International Universities Press.

Ehrenwald, J. 1974. "Out-of-the-Body Experiences and the Denial of Death." *Journal of Nervous and Mental Disease* 159:227–33.

Freud, S. 1900. "The Interpretation of Dreams." *S.E.* 4.

Greyson, B. 1983. "The Psychodynamics of Near-Death Experiences." *The Journal of Nervous and Mental Disease*. 171:376–81.

Honegger, B. 1979. Correspondence. *Parapsychology Review*. 10:24–26.

Jung, C. 1963. *Memories, Dreams, Reflections*. New York: Vintage.

Monroe, R. 1977. *Journeys Out of the Body*. Garden City, New York: Anchor Press/Doubleday.

Noyes, R. 1981. "The Subjective Response to Life Threatening Danger." Presented at the Annual Meeting of the American Psychiatric Association in New Orleans, Louisiana.

Palmer, J. 1978. "The Out-of-Body Experience: A Psychological Theory." *Parapsychology Review*. 9:19–22.

Rogo, D. 1982. "Psychological Models of the Out-of-Body Experience: A Review and Critical Evaluation." *Journal of Parapsychology*. 46:29–45.

Schafer, R. 1978. *Language and Insight*. New Haven: Yale University Press.

Sherwood, N. 1969. *The Logic of Explanation in Psychoanalysis.* New York: Academic Press.
Tolpin, M. 1974. "The Daedalus Experience: A Developmental Vicissitude of the Grandiose Fantasy." *The Annual of Psychoanalysis,* 2:213–28.
Twemlow, S.W., R. Hendren, G.O. Gabbard, F.C. Jones, and P. Norris. 1982. "Ego-Integrating Function of Psi States." *Journal of Psychiatric Treatment and Evaluation.* 4:41–49.
Waelder, R. 1930. "The Principle of Multiple Function: Observations on Overdetermination." In *Psychoanalysis: Observation, Theory and Application. Selected Papers of Robert Waelder,* edited by S. Guttman. New York: International Universities Press, 1976.

CHAPTER TWELVE

Bohm, D. 1980. *Wholeness and the Implicate Order.* London: Routledge and Kegan Paul.
Brain/Mind Bulletin. 1983. November 21, 9(1):1–2.
Brain/Mind Bulletin. 1983. October 24, 8(17):1.
Comfort, A. 1981. "The Implications of the Implicate." *Journal Soc. Biol. Struct.* 4:363–74.
Fox, O. (pseudonym). 1962. *Astral Projection: A Record of Out-of-the-Body Experiences.* Secaucus, NJ: University Books (originally published in 1939).
Hartwell, J., J. Janis, and S. Harary. 1975. "A Study of Physiological Variables Associated with Out-of-Body Experiences." *Research in Parapsychology—1974.* Metuchen, NJ: The Scarecrow Press, pp. 127–29.
Morris, R., S. Harary, J. Janis, J. Hartwell, and W. Roll. 1978. "Studies of Communication During Out-of-Body Experiences." *Journal of the American Society for Psychical Research* 72(1):1–21.
Osis, K., and J. Mitchell. 1977. "Physiological Correlates of Reported Out-of-Body Experiences." *Journal of the Society for Psychical Research* 49(772):525–36.
Palmer, J. 1979. "ESP and Out-of-Body Experiences: EEG Correlates." *Research in Parapsychology 1978.* Metuchen, NJ: The Scarecrow Press, pp. 135–38.
Rogo, D.S. 1984. "Researching the Out-of-the-Body Experience: The State of the Art." *Anabiosis* 4:21–49.
Rose, S. 1980. "Can the Neurosciences Explain the Mind." *Trends in Neurosciences* 3(5):1–4.
Salley, R.D. 1982. "REM Sleep During Out-of-Body Experiences." *Journal of the American Society for Psychical Research* 76:157–65.

Sherman, S. 1972. "Very Deep Hypnosis." *Journal of Transpersonal Psychology* 4(1):87–91.
Silverman, D. 1963. "Retrospective Study of the EEG in Coma." *Electroencephalography and Clinical Neurophysiology* 15:486–503.
Singer, J., and J. Antrobus. 1972. "Daydreaming, Imaginal Processes and Personality: A Normative Study." In *The Function and Nature of Imagery*, edited by P.W. Sheehan. New York: Academic Press, pp. 174–202.
Tart, C.T. 1968. "A Psychophysiological Study of Out-of-the-Body Experiences in a Selected Subject." *Journal of the American Society for Psychical Research* 62(7):3–27.
———. 1967. "A Second Psychophysiological Study of Out-of-the-Body Experiences in a Gifted Subject." *International Journal of Parapsychology* 9(4): 251–58.
Tellegan, A. 1976. Personal Communication.
Twemlow, S. 1977. "Epilogue: Personality File." In *Journeys Out of the Body*, edited by R.A. Monroe. New York: Anchor Press/Doubleday, pp. 175–80.
Wilber, K. 1980. *The Atman Project*. Wheaton, Ill.: The Theosophical Publishing House.

CHAPTER THIRTEEN

Becker, E. 1973. *The Denial of Death*. New York: The Free Press.
Blackmore, S. 1984. "Are Out-of-Body Experiences Evidence for Survival?" *Anabiosis* 3:137–55.
Brown, D. 1977. "Levels of Concentrative Meditation." *International Journal of Clinical and Experimental Hypnosis* 25:236–73.
Eccles, J. 1977. "The Human Person in Its Two-Way Relationship to the Brain." In *Research in Parapsychology—1976*. London: Scarecrow Press.
Edelheit, H. 1976. "Complementarity as a Rule in Psychological Research." *International Journal of Psycho-Analysis* 57:23–29.
Ellison, A. 1979. Personal Communication.
Erikson, E. 1962. "Reality and Actuality." *Journal of the American Psychoanalytic Association* 10:451–74.
Feigl, H. 1975. "Some Crucial Issues of Mind-Body Monism." In *Philosophical Aspects of the Mind-Body Problem*, edited by C. Cheng, pp. 22–34. Honolulu: The University Press of Hawaii.
Fox, O. (pseudonym). 1962. *Astral Projection: A Record of Out-of-the-Body Experiences*. Secaucus, NJ: University Books. (originally published in 1939.)
Gardner, M. 1981. "The Extraordinary Metal Bending of Professor Taylor."

In *Paranormal Borderlands of Science*, edited by K. Frazier, pp. 142–47. New York: Basic Books.
Globus, G. 1973a. "Consciousness and Brain: I. The Identity Thesis." *Archives of General Psychiatry* 29:153–60.
———. 1973b. "Consciousness and Brain: II. Introspection, the Qualia of Experience, and the Unconscious." *Archives of General Psychiatry* 29: 167–76.
Globus, G., and S. Franklin. 1980. "Prospects for the Scientific Observer of Perceptual Consciousness." In *The Psychobiology of Consciousness*, edited by J. Davidson and R. Davidson, pp. 465–81. New York: Plenum Press.
Grosso, M. 1976. "Some Varieties of Out-of-Body Experiences." *The Journal of the American Society for Psychical Research* 70:179–93.
Inglis, B. 1983. "Power Corrupts: Skepticism Corrodes. *A.S.P.R. Newsletter* 9(3):1-3.
Klein, G. 1973. "Two Theories or One?" *Bulletin of the Menninger Clinic* 37:102–32.
Maliszewski, M., S. Twemlow, D. Brown, and J. Engler. 1981. "A Phenomenological Typology of Intensive Meditation: A Suggested Methodology Using the Questionnaire Approach." *ReVision* 4:3–27.
Monroe, R. 1977. *Journeys Out of the Body*. New York: Anchor Doubleday.
Morris, R., S. Harary, J. Janis, J. Hartwell, and W. Roll. 1978. "Studies in Communication During Out-of-Body Experiences." *Journal of the American Society for Psychical Research* 72:1–22.
Muldoon, S., and H. Carrington. 1977. *The Projection of the Astral Body*. New York: Samuel Weiser. (originally published in 1929.)
Osis, K., and D. McCormick. 1980. "Kinetic Effects at the Ostensible Location of an Out-of-Body Projection during Perceptual Testing." *Journal of the American Society for Psychical Research* 74:319–29.
Oxford Dictionary of English Etymology, edited by C.T. Onions. 1966. Great Britain: Oxford at the Clarendon Press.
Polanyi, M. 1965. "The Structure of Consciousness." *Brain* 88:799–810.
Popper, K., and J. Eccles. 1977. *The Self and Its Brain*. New York: Springer International.
Rogo, D. 1984. "Researching the Out-of-Body Experience: the State of the Art." *Anabiosis* 4:21–49.
Rogo, D.S. 1978. *Mind Beyond the Body*. New York: Penguin Books Ltd.
Rosenthal, R. 1977. "Biasing Effects of Experimenters." *Et cetera* 34:253–64.
Rothstein, A. 1980. "Psychoanalytic Paradigms and their Narcissistic Investment." *Journal of the American Psychoanalytic Association* 28:385–95.
Sabom, M. 1982. *Recollections of Death*. New York: Harper and Row.
Salley, R.D. 1982. "REM Sleep during Out-of-Body Experiences." *Journal of the American Society for Psychical Research* 76:157–65.

Singer, B. 1981. "To Believe or Not to Believe." In *Science and the Paranormal*, edited by G.O. Abell and B. Singer, pp. 7–23. New York: Charles Scribner & Sons.

Stevenson, I. 1983. "Do We Need a New Word to Supplement 'Hallucination'?" *American Journal of Psychiatry* 140:1609–11.

Sulloway, I.J. 1979. *Freud, Biologist of the Mind*. New York: Basic Books.

Tart, C. 1972. "States of Consciousness and State Specific Sciences." *Science* 176:1203–10.

Trefil, J. 1983. "Grounds for Dismissal: Case Studies of the Rejection of Scientific Claims." *The Explorer* 1:8–9.

Wheelis, A. 1980. *The Scheme of Things*. New York: Harcourt Brace Jovanovich.

INDEX
NAME INDEX

Acker, B., 57
Adkins, J., 80
Alonso-Fernandez, F., 68
Ambrosino, S., 59
Angyal, A., 79
Antrobus, J.S., 112, 113, 210
Arkin, A.M., 102, 105
Arlow, J., 50
Aserinsky, E., 100
Atkinson, G., 150

Becker, C.B., 130, 139, 234
Becker, E., 196
Barber, T., 39
Beit-Hallahmi, B., 113
Bergler, E., 49
Bion, W., 72, 172
Blackmore, S.J., 5, 10, 12, 16, 20, 21, 24, 35, 109, 189, 223, 225, 226
Blank, H., 49
Blatt, S., 84, 86
Bliss, E.L., 114
Bogaert, L., 61
Bohm, D., 203
Brenner, C., 184
Broad, C.D., 4
Brown, D.P., 112, 237
Burton, A., 80
Bush, N., 160

Caine, R., 150
Caine, T.M., 28
Campbell, R., 169
Cardone, S., 91
Carr, D., 118, 130
Carrington, H., 6, 8, 104, 107
Castaneda, C., 106
Cayce, E., 10
Chapman, L., 82
Chattah, L., 169
Clauzure, G., 220
Cleveland, S., 80, 81
Coleman, S., 63

Comfort, A., 203
Coyne, L., 124
Crookall, R., 15, 20, 22–23, 25, 107, 108

Damas Mora, J., 67, 68, 69
Darby, J., 92
Davidson, R., 151
de Saint-Denys, H., 108
Descartes, R., 233
Dewhurst, K., 63, 69
Dickstein, L.S., 28, 151
Dillon, D., 80
Dobson, M., 142
Druss, R., 142

Eastman, M., 16
Eccles, J., 233
Edelheit, H., 233
Ehrenwald, J., 5, 133, 188
Eidelberg, L., 49
Ellison, A., 226
Erikson, E., 227
Eysenck, H., 150
Eysenck, S.B.G., 28, 150

Faguet, R., 68, 71, 76
Faraday, A., 106
Federn, P., 50, 81, 83, 105, 170–172, 173–174, 180–181, 182
Feigl, H., 235
Fenichel, O., 48
Fisher, S., 47, 80, 81
Foulkes, D., 102–103, 116
Fox, O., 6, 8, 103–104, 105, 107, 220, 224, 225
Freedman, N., 91, 114, 116
Freeman, T., 78, 86
Freud, S., 48, 70, 72, 83, 103, 113, 169–170, 69, 173, 180, 185, 187, 196, 201
Friedman, H., 149

Gabbard, G.O., 32, 46, 47, 50–51, 57, 86, 124, 136, 142, 180
Gackenbach, J.I., 108
Gallup, G., 125–126, 129, 143
Gardner, M., 225
Gazzaniga, M., 72
Giambra, L.M., 111
Giovetti, P., 36
Globus, G., 235
Goertzel, V., 92
Gordon, R., 117
Grand, S., 85
Green, C.E., 9, 12, 13, 16, 17, 20–21, 23, 24, 25, 35, 75, 103, 107, 142
Green, J., 143–144
Greyson, B., 118, 124, 125, 133–134, 136, 138, 142, 143, 151, 152, 188
Grinberg, L., 172
Grof, S., 129, 152
Grosso, M., 128, 130, 134, 235
Grotstein, J., 63, 71–73, 76, 112

Hamersma, R., 80
Hamilton, J., 63–64
Haraldsson, E., 10, 12, 135, 152
Harary, S., 103, 205–206, 208
Hariton, E.B., 113
Harrow, M., 47, 81–82
Hart, H., 8, 12, 20
Hartwell, J., 205
Hill, H., 229
Hill, J.A., 8
Hinsie, L., 169
Holtzman, W., 81
Honegger, B., 189
Hood, R.W., 33
Horowitz, J.M., 112, 238

Inglis, B., 231–232
Irwin, H.J., 12, 16, 32, 39, 101, 111, 151
Isaacs, D., 112
Isakower, O., 116

James, W., 6, 25, 107, 111
Jacobson, E., 49
Jenkins, S., 91
Jones, F.C., 27, 46, 124, 207

Jung, C., 188

Kant, E., 222
Katan, M., 72
Kennedy, R.B., Jr., 28, 45
Khemka, K., 162
Klein, G., 228–229
Kleitman, N., 102
Kletti, R., 51, 57, 124, 132, 142–143
Klinger, E., 111
Kohr, R.L., 10, 12
Kohut, H., 51, 152, 165, 171
Kokonis, N., 81
Kramer, M., 101
Kreutziger, S., 124

LaBerge, S.P., 107, 108, 109, 110
Lancaster, N., 79
Leaning, F.E., 115
LeDoux, J., 72
Lhermitte, J., 61, 62, 63, 66
Lidz, T., 81
Lindley, J., 143, 146
Lukianowicz, N., 61, 66–67, 68–70, 71, 73–74, 76, 79, 89–90, 91, 92, 239
Lundahl, C., 139
Lunn, V., 74

McCormick, D., 223
McDevitt, J., 179
McHarg, J.F., 130
McKellar, P., 115, 116
McVaughn, M.R., 8
Mahler, M., 84, 179
Maliszewski, M., 40, 237
Mantegazza, P., 92–93
Maslow, A.H., 25
Maury, L.F.A., 114
Mauskopf, S.H., 8
Menninger-Lerchenthal, E., 62, 68
Miller, N., 231
Monroe, R.A., 6, 7, 29, 31, 107, 190, 191–192, 194, 205, 207–209, 220, 223
Moody, R.A., Jr., 123–124, 125, 132, 138, 156, 162
Morris, R.L., 103, 205, 223
Morse, M., 160–161

Muldoon, S., 6, 8, 104, 107
Murdock, G.P., 11
Myers, F.W.H., 8, 114
Myers, S., 10, 12, 32–33
Myers, W., 50

Nemiah, J., 47, 57, 58–59
Noyes, R., 46, 51, 57–58, 125, 131–132, 139, 142–143, 188
Nunberg, H., 48

Olson, R., 91
Osis, K., 4, 13, 25, 35, 36, 135, 204, 206–207, 223
Ostow, N., 70, 76

Palmer, J., 4, 5, 9, 10, 12, 16, 39, 109, 151, 189, 206
Papson, D., 80
Pearson, J., 69
Pivik, T., 102
Polanyi, M., 226
Pope, K.S., 111
Popper, K., 233

Quay, H.D., 32
Quinlan, D., 47, 82

Rank, O., 62, 63, 65, 69–70
Richard, J.T., 114
Richardson, A., 112, 113–114
Richet, C., 232
Ring, K., 124, 126, 129, 131, 138, 139–140, 151–152
Rinsley, D., 172, 174
Roberts, W., 57
Rodin, E.A., 130, 143
Rogo, D.S., 3, 23, 188, 204, 223, 225
Rose, S., 203
Rosen, D., 142
Rosenfeld, H., 49
Rosenthal, R., 228, 230–231
Rothstein, A., 229
Rubin, J., 149

Sabom, M., 46, 74, 124, 131, 135, 143, 151–152, 223, 224
Sadock, B., 116, 117
Sagan, C., 129–130
Salley, R.D., 103, 204, 230
Sambroski, A., 91
Sandler, J., 163
Sarlin, C., 49
Satre, J., 172
Schafer, R., 163, 187
Schilder, P., 48, 81, 178
Schlaugh, R., 116
Schwarz, J., 153
Seidner, R., 47, 80
Selinsky, H., 57
Shannon, P., 203
Shapiro, D., 111
Sharpe, E.F., 105
Sherman, S., 220–221
Sherwood, N., 185
Shiels, D., 11, 16, 111
Shulka, T., 79
Siegel, R.K., 101, 131, 143, 152
Silverman, D., 220
Simpson, L., 115
Singer, J.L., 111, 113, 210, 224
Smith, P., 16–17
Smith, S., 152, 164
Snyder, F., 103
Sollier, P., 61, 66
Sommer, R., 80
Sparrow, G.S., 107
Stamm, J., 49
Starker, S., 111, 116
Stevenson, I., 124, 125, 138, 142, 239
Stolorow, R., 50, 51
Sulloway, I.J., 233
Swann, Ingo, 206, 207, 208–209

Tart, C.T., 5, 11, 12–13, 17, 103, 204–205, 208, 228, 236
Tausk, V., 73, 83
Taylor, J.G., 225
Tellegen, A., 39, 101, 150, 210
Thale, T., 114
Tolstoy, L., 191
Tolpin, M., 190–191
Traub, A., 82
Trefil, J., 229
Tucker, G., 47
Twemlow, S.W., 3, 14, 32, 46, 103, 112, 124, 136, 149, 194, 207

Van Eeden, F., 105
Vassar, C., 16
Vernon, J.A., 114

Waelder, R., 51–52, 202
Walsh, R., 27
Weckowicz, T., 80
Wheelis, A., 240
Whiteman, J.H.M., 5, 107

Wigan, A., 69
Wilber, K., 220
Wild, C., 84, 86
Wilson, S., 39

Yalom, I., 164
Yram, 8

Zorick, F.J., 116

SUBJECT INDEX

"Absorption" scale, 28, 32–33, 37, 146, 150, 151, 194; in college students, 32; in dream OBE subjects, 32; need for achievement and, 32; neuroticism and, 32; religiosity and, 32 (*see also* mental health of OBE subjects); verbalizing tendency, 32; visualizing tendency, 32
actuality (as defined by Erikson), 230
"after-death" experience, 132, 153
age range of OBE subjects, 34–35, 36
alpha-methyldopa, 92–93, 239
altered mind/body perception, 3, 45, 74–75, 78, 80, 92, 123, 169, 170, 175–176, 179, 222
altered state of consciousness, 5, 95, 189, 228, 236, 238–240
alternative natural explanations of OBE percepts, 224, 229–230
anesthesia, 150, 153
antipsychotic medication: as a cause of OBE, 92, 239; in depression, 55, 59; in schizophrenic body boundary disturbances, 87–88, 159–160
astral body, 178
astral catalepsy, 105
astral projection, 201
autophany, 75–76
attentional shift, 236–237
autoscopic hallucinations (*see* autoscopy)
autoscopic phenomena (*see* autoscopy)
autoscopy, 60–77; "autoscopic near-death experiences," 74; case examples, 65–67, 68; characteristics, 67; as a clinical syndrome, 66–68; and the conscience, 70; as defensive reassurance against death, 70; definition, 61; as a form of altered mind/body perception, 74–75, 175–176; diagnostic differentiation from OBE, 74–76; idiopathic, 70, 76; "interhemispheric diplopia" in, 72; kinesthetic perception in, 66–67; as a literary theme, 61–66; and migraines, 67; organic causes of, 68–69; projective identification in, 71–72, 74; psychological causes of, 69–74; restitutive function of, 71; and seizure disorders, 67; splitting in, 70, 71, 72, 73; treatment of, 76–77 (*see also* double, doppelgänger)

bardo, 220 (*see also* electroencephographic correlates of OBE)
"before-death" experience, 132, 151, 153
being of light, 124, 125, 127, 130, 131, 136, 141, 159, 160, 162–166
belief system, 227
blood volume in OBE, 207
Body Ego Technique (BET), 92
bodily ego: in Federn, 171–175, 176–182, 238–239; in Freud, 83, 171–172; in schizophrenia, 85–86
body image, 177–178, 188
body scheme, 177–179, 238–239
borderline personality disorder, 47–48, 55, 199–200, 294–98
"buoyancy," 172

castration anxiety, 50, 52
clairvoyance, 224
cocaine intoxication, 92–93
"cognitive map," 189, 226
cognitive-perceptual style, 151, 153
community college students, 29, 30–31
context of the near-death experience, 139–153; "Absorption," 146, 150–151; anesthesia, 153; anesthetic cluster, 150; cardiac arrest cluster, 150; cognitive-perceptual style, 151, 153; demographic factors, 144–145, 151; drug usage, 145, 152; emotional stress cluster, 149–150; intoxicant cluster, 150; low-stress cluster, 149; multivariate analysis, 149–150; pre-existing medical conditions, 145–146, 152, 153; psychological health, 146; univariate analysis, 144–148
continuum of altered mind/body perception, 175–183

cultural programming, 128–129, 161–162

"Daedalus experience," 190–191
danger-seeking scale, 28, 32, 150 (*see also* mental health of OBE subjects)
daydreams, 94–95, 110–114; in borderline patients, 112; in aging, 112; arousing function, 112–113; compared to OBE, 112; correlation with cognitive and personality attitudes, 112; cultural influences, 111; definition, 111–112; relation to psychiatric illness, 111; types, 111–112; visual style, 112; wishfulfilling qualities, 113
Death Anxiety Scale, 150, 192
death: attitudes toward, 28 (*see also* mental health of OBE subjects)
decline effect, 231–232
deja vu, 47
demographic characteristics of OBE subjects, 34–41 (*see also* age range, education, drug and alcohol use, hypnosis, income category, marital status, meditation, religion, sex difference)
denial of death, 70, 133, 158, 192, 193, 194, 195, 196, 234–235
dental anesthesia, 173
depersonalization, 45–59; and accidents, 47, 51; and castration anxiety, 50; and diagnostic category, 47; and disintegration anxiety, 51; and self-mutilation, 48, 52–53; and separation- individuation, 50; and stage fright, 47, 50–51; as a defense against and exhibitionism, 49; at the acropolis, 48; definition, 46–47; in the "Wolf Man," 48; psychological theories of, 48–51; "self- induced," 28–40
derealization, 46, 47, 179
design errors, 225
Differential Personality Questionnaire, 28, 210 (*see also* mental health of OBE subjects)
discrediting of researcher, 225

disintegration anxiety, 51
dissociation, of bodily and mental ego, 174–175, 176, 182, 239–240
doppelgänger, 60, 64, 188 (*see also* double, autoscopy)
double, the: and Bertrand Russell, 63–64; and guardian spirits, 62; and Joseph Conrad, 63–64; historical origins of, 61–66; as a literary theme, 61–66; and narcissistic transferences, 64; and Narcissus, 63; in *The Picture of Dorian Gray*, 64; and the shadow, 62; and the soul, 62–63
Draw-a-Person Test, 81
dream OBE, 94, 96, 100–101; Absorption score in, 101; descriptive features, 100; flying and falling dream OBE, 95; influence of toxic/metabolic stimuli, 101–102; similarity to NDE, 100
dreams and dissociation of bodily and mental ego, 174, 179–180; of flying, 198, 201; as normal mental activities, 187; overdetermination in, 186–187
drug and alcohol use in OBE subjects, 39

education of OBE subjects, 35–36
ego atony, 181
ego boundary: in Federn, 172–175, 176–183; in Freud, 173; loss of in NDE, 133; origin of concept, 83; in schizophrenia, 78, 83–86
ego cathexis: bodily and mental, 173–175, 176–182, 228, 238–239; in schizophrenia, 83
ego feeling, 171, 175, 176, 182
"ego homeostasis" model, 189
ego ideal, 141
ego-integrating function, 193–194, 200
ego-uncoupling model, 238–240
electroencephalogic correlates of OBE: alphoid state, 205; anxiety during, 210; barometric pressure during, 210; in coma, 220; correlation with ESP, 206; deep hypnosis, 220–221; influence of medication, 220; interhemispheric differences, 208; literature review, 204–207; OBE

wave shape, 219; power spectral analysis, 208; in relation to REM stages, 205; in relation to sleep stages, 205; relative humidity during, 210; in Robert Monroe, 207–208; room temperature, 210
Er: story of, 142
estrangement, 46, 50, 52, 238 (*see also* depersonalization)
engram, 178
existential dread, 196, 234–235
experimenter bias, 230–232
explanatory usefulness of percept, 227, 228–229
"extrapsychic" perception, 135, 224

Fourier transformation, 210

Galvanic Skin Resistance in OBE, 207
"Golden Fantasy," 152, 164
grandiose self, 64, 152

hallucination and OBE, 239
hallucinogens, 92–93, 130–131, 182–183, 228, 236, 239
Hamlet, 227
heart rate in OBE, 205
heautoscopy (*see* autoscopy)
hypnagogic state, 95, 113–118; body image disturbances in, 117; compared to hallucinations, 117–118; compared to hypnopompic, 114–115; compared to OBE, 115; in depression, 116; descriptive features, 113–115; ego functions in, 116; electroencephalographic correlates, 115–116; in hysteria, 116; Isakower phenomena in, 116; in narcolepsy, 116; in NDEs, 118; prevalence, 115; relation to IQ, 115; relation to personality features, 115–116; relation to social class, 115; sex differences, 115; in tricyclic antidepressants, 116; visual versus auditory features, 113–115
hypnosis: experience of in OBE subjects, 38, 39–40; relationship to Absorption scale, 39–40

hypnopompic state, 95; general feature, 113–118; subvocalizations in, 117 (*see also* hypnagogic state)
Hysteroid scale, 28, 32, 150 (*see also* mental health of OBE subjects)

Imaginal Process Inventory, 210–211; in OBE subjects, 211
immortality wish, 70, 133, 188, 193, 195, 234–235
incestuous sexuality, 52–53, 54–55, 195–196, 197
income category of OBE subjects, 34, 35–36
International Association for Near-Death Studies, 160
Isakower phenomenon, 95, 116

jamais vu, 47

laboratory experiments with gifted subjects, 222–225, 230–232
"location-effect," 232
LSD, 129–130, 153, 228, 236 (*see also* hallucinogens)
lucid dream, 95, 105–110; anxiety in, 109; awareness of body in, 107; compared to OBE, 107–110; definition, 105; descriptive features, 107; electroencephalographic findings in, 109; field independence in, 108; in flying and falling dreams, 109; mental imagery in, 109; mystical qualities in, 107; neuroticism in, 109; in relation to frequency of dream recall, 109; surveys of, 109

M5000 trainees, 29, 30–31
marital status of OBE subjects, 34–36
medial ego feeling, 171–175
meditation: association with OBE, 40; attentional shift in, 236–237 decathexis of bodily ego in, 176; frequency of in OBE subjects, 38, 40; idiosyncratic techniques, 40; in OBE subjects, 38, 40; Transcendental, 29, 30–32
mental ego, 169–175, 176–182

mental health of OBE subjects, 30–34;
  Absorption, 32; alcohol and drug use,
  30–31; child interpersonal
  relationships, 31; close adult
  interpersonal relationships, 31;
  danger seeking, 32; death anxiety, 32;
  income management, 30–31;
  negative emotions, 31–32;
  psychological well-being, 31–32;
  psychosomatic symptoms, 31–32 (see
  also Absorption scale, attitudes to
  death, Danger-seeking scale,
  demographic characteristics of OBE
  subjects, Hysteroid scale,
  Psychoticism scale)
mescaline (see hallucinogens)
metapsychology, 169–183, definition,
  169–170
methodological errors, 224–225
migraine: aura, 239; and autoscopy, 67
mind-body problem (see philosophy and
  OBE)
Monroe Institute of Applied Sciences,
  190
Monroe, Robert: case of, 190–192,
  207–208 (see also electroencephographic correlates of OBE)
multiple causation, 185–186, 194, 202,
  239
mystical experiences: in lucid dreams,
  107; personality correlates of, 33 (see
  also demographic characteristics of
  OBE subjects; impact of experience;
  OBE, religion)

narcissistic investment in a paradigm,
  229–230
narcissistic transferences, 64; alter ego,
  64; twinship, 64
near-death experience, 123–166;
  "archetype of death," 134; attitudinal
  and belief changes, 125, 128, 138;
  being of light, 124–125, 127, 130,
  131, 136, 141, 158–159, 160–161,
  162–166; birth models, 129–130;
  case examples, 126–127, 140–141,
  154–159; in children, 154–166;
  context of, 139–153; cultural
  programming, 128–129, 161–162;
  differentiation from OBE, 136–138;
  explanatory hypotheses for, 127–136;
  "extrapsychic" perception, 135; fivestage continuum, 124–125; incidence
  of, 124–125–126; Moody's
  composite experience, 123–124;
  neurophysiological models,
  130–131; overview of, 123–138;
  panoramic memory, 123, 124, 125, 134,
  136, 138, 161, 164 ; paranormal
  models, 134–136; psychological
  models, 131–133; and religious
  beliefs, 125, 145, 151–152;
  review of literature, 124–126;
  survival hypothesis, 134–135
nightmares, 94

object constancy, 51
occupational groups of OBE subjects,
  35–36
oedipus complex, 48, 227
out-of-body experience: case examples,
  177, 185–186, 196–202; causation
  and meaning, 184–202, 239–240;
  defensive function of, 197–198;
  definition of, 3–8; differentiation
  from autoscopy, 74–76;
  differentiation from
  depersonalization, 56–59, 197–198;
  differentiation from hallucinations,
  239; differentiation from NDE,
  136–138; differentiation from
  schizophrenic body boundary
  disturbances, 89–91; ego functions in,
  25–26; metapsychology of,
  175–;183; phenomenological
  prototype, 26; psychological/
  demographic prototype, 40–41;
  questionnaire survey methodology,
  15, 25–26; reality in, 225–232, 238–
  239; review of psychological theories,
  188–190; taxonomy of, 5–8
out-of-body experience—impact,
  23–25; autonomy, 25; belief in
  survival after death, 22, 24; closure on
  existential questions, 24; fear, 24;
  negative affective responses, 24–25;

positive affective responses, 23–24; religious experience, 24, 25
out-of-body experience—incidence, 8–13; anthropological survey, 11; in college students, 8–9, 10; in marijuana users, 12; random surveys, 9–10; special interest groups, 10, 13; spontaneous cases, 8
out-of-body experience—phenomenology, 14, 19–23; consciousness remaining within the body, 25–26; dream qualities, 22–23; energy, 21; features in top 25%, 19–20; form similar to physical body, 21; nonphysical beings, 21; silver cord, 20; sounds, 22–23; surrounding environment, 21; tunnel experience, 21; vibrations, 21
out-of-body experience—preexisting conditions, 15–19; belief systems and, 16–17; while dreaming, 17; effect of drug use, 17; motive for seeking OBE, 18; when near death, 18; by number of OBEs reported, 17; surveys of, 14–16; type of emotional stress, 17–18
overdetermination, 51–52, 186–187, 194, 197, 201, 202, 239

PAL—Profile of Adaptation to Life Questionnaire, 14; demographic characteristic of groups, 34–36; PAL scales, 29–30; reliability and validity, 29; strengths, 30–31; subjects use, 29 (*see also* mental health of OBE subjects, questionnaire survey methodology)
panoramic memory, 123–124, 125, 138, 161, 163, 164
pananormal explanations, 134–136, 223–224
participatory reality, 225–232
preexisting conditions: in NDE, 139–153; in OBE, 14–18 (*see also* context of the near-death experience)
phantom limb phenomenon, 178–179
"phenomenal I," 234
philosophy and OBE, 230–235; attentional shift, 236–237; Descartes, 233; dualism, 233–236, 238; hypophenomenalism, 235; identity thesis, 235; interactionism, 233; monism, 235; parallelism, 233; "phenomenal I," 236–237
POBE—Profile of Out-of-Body Experience questionnaire, 14, 28 (*see also* OBE questionnaire survey methodology)
"pre-reflective cogito," 172
professional conference attendees, 29, 30–32
"proto-thoughts," 172
psychiatric outpatients, 29, 30–32
psychic determinism, 184–185
psychokinesis, 224
Psychoticism scale, 28, 32, 150 (*see also* mental health of OBE subjects)

reality in the OBE (*see* participatory reality)
reality testing, 181–182
rebirth, 70, 200
religion, 36–39; current religion, 36; interest in religion, 36, 37–39; interpretation of OBE, 37–39; in multiple OBE subjects, 37; religious background, 36, 37
REM dream, 94–95, 101–103; awareness of body in, 104; compared to OBE, 103–105, definition of, 102–103; imagery in, 103–104; physiology, 103 (*see also* EEG changes in OBE)
respiration rate in OBE, 206, 207
retrospective verification of OBE percepts, 135, 222–225
Rorschach responses: in OBE subjects, 192, 200; in phantom limb patients, 179; in schizophrenic body boundary disturbances, 81–82

schizophrenia, 78, 201–202 (*see also* schizophrenic body boundary disturbances)
schizophrenic body boundary disturbances, 78–93; categories of, 80; clinical manifestations of, 79–82;

developmental understanding, 82–86; differentiation from OBE, 89–91; and "fusion" phenomena, 80, 86; incidences of, 79–80; metapsychology of, 181–182; review of studies, 79–82; Rorschach responses in, 81–82; treatment of, 91–93
seizures, temporal lobe, 239
self-esteem, 163–164
self-mutilation, 47–48, 52–53
separation anxiety, 200–201
separation hypothesis, 3, 204, 222–240
separation-individuation, 50, 199–200
sex differences in OBE, 34–36
shadow, 62
soul, 62–63, 70, 134–135, 193, 194, 234
splitting: in autoscopy, 70, 71–72, 73; in the doubling phenomenon, 65; in depersonalization, 46–47, 49–50, 53, 56–57; in OBE subject, 201
stage fright, 47, 50–51
state of consciousness: altered, 5, 127–128, 189, 228, 236, 238–239; as determinant of reality, 227–228
superego, 141, 163–164, 165–166
survival hypothesis, 134–135
synesthesia, 228

telepathy, 224
transference: Einstein as transference figure, 229; and meaning of OBE, 196; narcissistic, 64; objects, 163, 164; and reality perception, 226–227
transitional states in OBE, 208–209
treatment: of autoscopy, 76–77; of depersonalization, 59; of schizophrenic body boundary disturbances, 91–93
tunnel experience, 125, 127, 130, 131, 136, 140–141, 158–161

window in consciousness, 219–220 (*see also* electroencephalographic correlates of OBE)
"witness effect," 232

"Y," Miss: case methodology, 209–211; description of OBE, 212–219; electroencephalographic findings, 219–220; imagery correlates, 210–211; in relation to psychic trauma, 219–220; personality correlates, 210–211 (*see also* Differential Personality Questionnaire, electroencephalographic correlates of OBE, Imaginal Process Inventory)

ABOUT THE AUTHORS

Glen O. Gabbard, M.D., is Staff Psychiatrist and Psychoanalyst, The Menninger Foundation, and Section Chief, C. F. Menninger Memorial Hospital, Topeka, Kansas. He is also a faculty member of the Topeka Institute for Psychoanalysis and the Karl Menninger School of Psychiatry.

Dr. Gabbard has published widely in diverse areas of psychiatry and psychoanalysis. His articles have appeared in the *International Journal of Psycho-Analysis, Journal of the American Psychoanalytic Association, American Journal of Psychiatry, Psychiatry*, and *Journal of Nervous and Mental Disease.*

Dr. Gabbard holds the M.D. degree from Rush Medical College, Chicago, Illinois, and is a graduate of the Karl Menninger School of Psychiatry and the Topeka Institute for Psychoanalysis.

Stuart W. Twemlow, M.D., is in the private practice of psychiatry in Topeka, Kansas. He is Clinical Associate Professor of Psychiatry, University of Kansas School of Medicine, Kansas City, Kansas, and Teaching Associate, Topeka Institute for Psychoanalysis, Topeka, Kansas.

Dr. Twemlow has published widely in the fields of altered states of consciousness and clinical psychiatry. His publications have appeared in *American Journal of Psychiatry, Journal of Consulting and Clinical Psychology, Journal of Nervous and Mental Disease, Psychiatry*, and *Psychotherapy: Theory, Research, and Practice.*

Dr. Twemlow holds a M.B.Ch.B. from the University of Otago Medical School, Dunedin, New Zealand. He is also a graduate of the Karl Menninger School of Psychiatry and an advanced candidate in the Topeka Institute for Psychoanalysis. Dr. Twemlow holds a Black Belt in Kaju Kempo Karate and in the Okinawan Kobudo (Weapons) System.

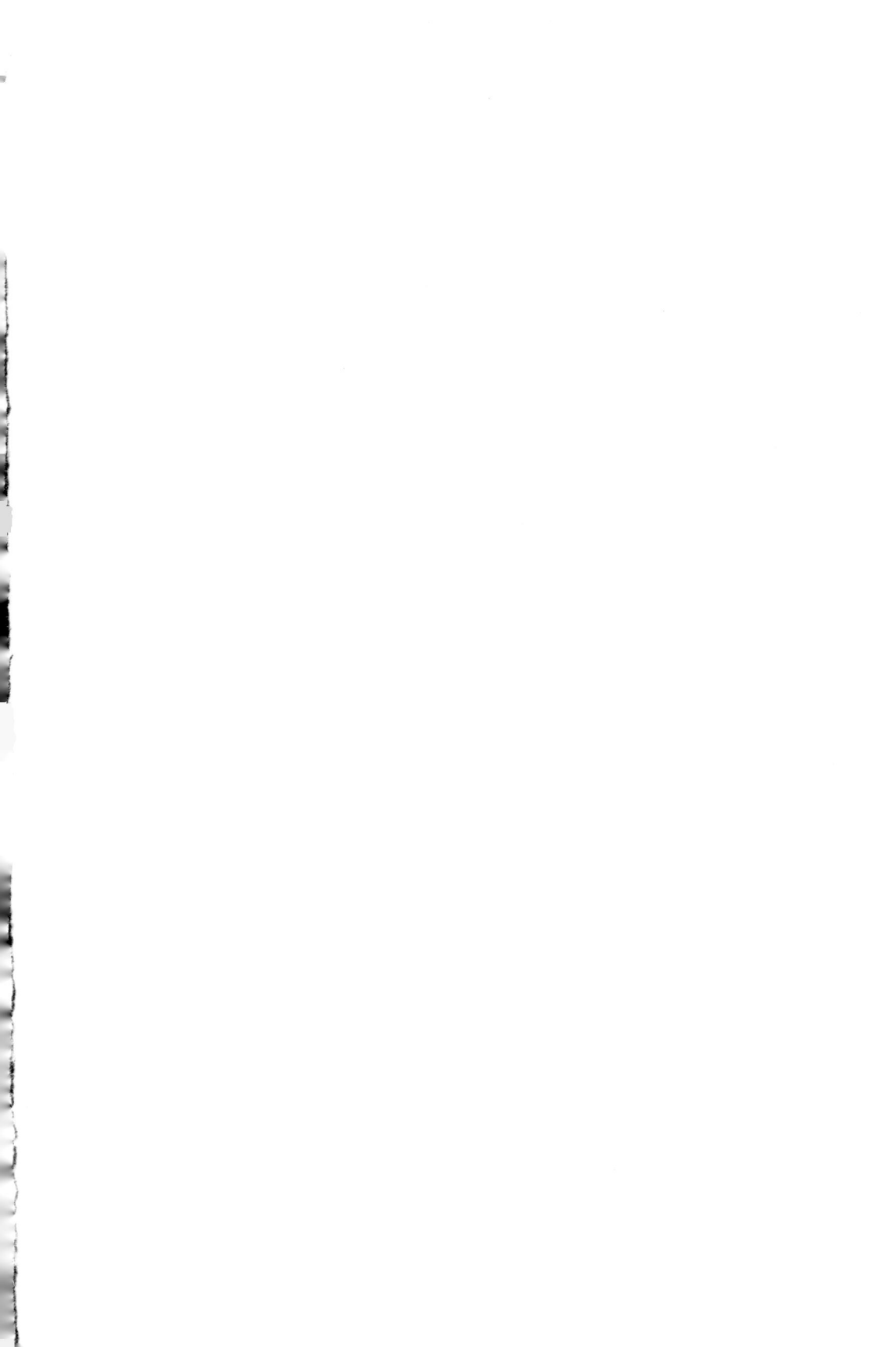